UNRAVELING ALZHEIMER'S
The Definitive Guide to Its Cause and Cure

Pietro Paolo

Copyright © 2024 by Pietro Paolo
All rights reserved.
No part of this book may be reproduced in any form
or by any means, including electronic or mechanical,
without the prior written permission of the publisher,
except for brief quotations in printed reviews.

ISBN: 9798305401097
Cover design by Pietro Paolo
Printed in USA

Foreword	9
A Personal Connection to Alzheimer's	9
The Journey Toward Clarity	11
Introduction	13
Why Alzheimer's Remains a Mystery	13
The Stakes: Humanity's Greatest Cognitive Challenge	16
A Breakthrough in Understanding	19
Part I: The Origins of Alzheimer's Disease	22
Chapter 1: The History of Alzheimer's	22
From Alois Alzheimer to Modern Research	22
Missteps and Breakthroughs Over the Decades	24
Chapter 2: The Biology of Memory and Brain Aging	27
Understanding the Healthy Brain	27
How Aging Impacts Neurological Function	29
Chapter 3: Plaques, Tangles, and Beyond	32
The Amyloid Cascade Hypothesis	32
Tau Tangles: A Closer Look	34
Revisiting the Role of Neuroinflammation	36
Chapter 4: The Missing Puzzle Piece	39
The Role of Mitochondrial Dysfunction	39
Environmental Triggers and Lifestyle Factors	41
Genetics vs. Epigenetics	44
Chapter 5: Root Cause Revealed	48
Synthesizing Decades of Evidence	48
The Central Role of Chronic Inflammation	50
Part II: The Cure for Alzheimer's Disease	54
Chapter 6: The Holistic Approach to Healing	54

Why One-Size-Fits-All Treatments Fail	54
Tailoring Solutions to Individual Needs	57
Chapter 7: Breakthrough Therapies	61
Targeting Amyloid and Tau Pathways	61
The Role of Anti-Inflammatory Drugs	64
Cutting-Edge Gene Therapy	67
Chapter 8: The Nutritional Connection	72
Diet's Role in Brain Health	72
Nutraceuticals That Support Cognitive Function	75
The Ketogenic Diet and Beyond	80
Chapter 9: Restoring the Brain's Ecosystem	84
Gut-Brain Axis: The Forgotten Frontier	84
Detoxifying the Brain: The Role of Sleep and Glymphatic Drainage	87
Supporting Neurogenesis	91
Chapter 10: Lifestyle Medicine	95
Exercise as Medicine for the Brain	95
Stress Reduction and Mindfulness	98
Social Engagement and Cognitive Resilience	102
Part III: Preventing Alzheimer's	106
Chapter 11: Risk Reduction Strategies	106
Early Detection and Biomarkers	106
Personalized Preventative Plans	110
Chapter 12: Building a Brain-Healthy World	114
Policies for Public Health	114
Educating the Next Generation	117
Part IV: The Future of Alzheimer's Research	121

Chapter 13: Bridging Gaps in Science	121
What We Still Don't Know	121
Collaborative Science and Open-Source Data	125
Chapter 14: A Vision for the Future	130
Toward a World Without Alzheimer's	130
Expanding the Cure to Other Neurological Diseases	133
Conclusion	138
Why This Matters for Humanity	138
A Call to Action	141
Appendices	144
Glossary of Terms	144
Summary of Key Studies	149
Practical Guides for Caregivers and Patients	154

Foreword

A Personal Connection to Alzheimer's

The first time I truly understood the devastating impact of Alzheimer's disease, it wasn't through a textbook or a clinical study. It was through the eyes of someone I loved. My grandmother, once a vibrant and fiercely independent woman, began to forget small things—a misplaced set of keys, the name of a neighbor she'd known for years. At first, it seemed like the normal signs of aging, the kind we all shrug off as harmless. But then, the gaps in her memory grew larger, like fractures in a once-solid foundation.

Soon, she couldn't remember my name, the sound of her laughter quieted, and the person who had been a pillar of strength for our family became lost in a fog of confusion. Watching her struggle with the simplest tasks was heartbreaking, but what hurt the most was seeing the fear in her eyes when she realized something was slipping away—something she couldn't control or stop.

Her diagnosis of Alzheimer's disease came like a storm, sudden and overwhelming. It wasn't just a medical term; it was a sentence. And while doctors offered treatments that might slow its progression, there was no cure, no promise of a future where her mind would remain her own. As I grappled with the helplessness of the situation, I made a promise—to her, to myself, and to the countless others facing the same battle—that I would dedicate my life to understanding this disease and finding a way to end its relentless grip on humanity.

This promise became my guiding light, pushing me through years of research, countless late nights, and moments of doubt. Alzheimer's is more than a disease that robs individuals of their memories; it steals the essence of who they are and leaves families grieving the loss of someone still physically present.

But amid the heartbreak, I discovered something extraordinary: hope. Hope in the resilience of the human spirit, in the brilliance of scientific minds working tirelessly, and in the possibility of a future where Alzheimer's is no longer a source of fear but a conquered foe.

This book is the culmination of that journey. It is a roadmap born of my personal experiences, rigorous analysis of the data, and an unwavering belief that answers exist if we are willing to seek them. My grandmother's story is one of millions, but her legacy lives on in these pages. She taught me that love and determination can fuel even the most daunting quests.

To those who have watched a loved one slip away, who have felt the weight of this disease in their lives, and who dare to dream of a cure: this book is for you. Together, we can honor the memories of those we've lost by building a future where Alzheimer's is no longer a part of the human experience.

With gratitude and determination,

Pietro Paolo

The Journey Toward Clarity

Alzheimer's disease has often been described as a puzzle, its pieces scattered across the vast landscapes of biology, genetics, and neuroscience. For much of my career, I felt like a determined yet frustrated traveler, navigating this complex terrain without a clear map. The journey was filled with moments of discovery, dead ends, and an unshakable sense of urgency.

What sets Alzheimer's apart from many other diseases is its sheer complexity. It is not a single, isolated problem with an obvious solution but a cascade of interconnected processes that impact the very core of what makes us human: our memory, identity, and relationships. Every researcher, clinician, and caregiver involved in this battle understands the weight of this challenge.

When I first embarked on this journey, the prevailing theories seemed promising but incomplete. The focus on amyloid plaques and tau tangles dominated the field, but the more I delved into the data, the more I realized how much remained unexplained. Why did some people with significant amyloid buildup never develop cognitive decline? Why did certain lifestyle factors appear to offer protection while others accelerated the disease? The deeper I looked, the clearer it became that we were missing critical pieces of the puzzle.

The turning point came not from a single revelation but from a shift in perspective. Instead of trying to isolate one cause or one cure, I began to think holistically. What if Alzheimer's was not just a disease of the brain but a systemic condition—one influenced by inflammation, metabolic health, and the interplay of genetics and environment? This broader view opened doors to new hypotheses and collaborative research that crossed disciplines.

The journey toward clarity also required humility. I had to question long-held assumptions, admit when data contradicted my expectations, and embrace the uncertainty that comes with scientific discovery. But these moments of doubt often led to the most significant breakthroughs. Each step forward, no matter how small, brought me closer to understanding the intricate mechanisms driving this disease.

This book represents the culmination of that journey—not just my own but the collective effort of countless researchers, clinicians, and caregivers who have contributed to this field. It is a testament to the power of persistence, the importance of questioning the status quo, and the profound impact of working together toward a common goal.

Clarity does not mean we have all the answers, but it means we are finally asking the right questions. It means we are closer than ever to unraveling the mysteries of Alzheimer's and finding a path toward prevention, treatment, and ultimately, a cure.

For those who are just beginning their own journey—whether as a caregiver, a patient, or an advocate—I hope this book provides the guidance and hope you need. For those who have been walking this path alongside me, let us continue forward, fueled by the knowledge that every step brings us closer to the day when Alzheimer's is a chapter in history, not a sentence in someone's future.

With clarity comes hope, and with hope, anything is possible.
Pietro Paolo

Introduction

Why Alzheimer's Remains a Mystery

For more than a century, Alzheimer's disease has perplexed scientists, physicians, and families alike. Despite immense advances in medical technology and research, this condition remains one of the most enigmatic and devastating illnesses known to humanity. What makes Alzheimer's particularly elusive is not just its complexity but the way it challenges our understanding of the brain, aging, and disease itself.

At its core, Alzheimer's is a disorder of memory—a process we often take for granted but that defines who we are. Yet, the precise mechanisms behind memory loss, the formation of amyloid plaques and tau tangles, and the eventual breakdown of cognitive functions remain partially veiled in mystery. For decades, researchers have diligently sought answers, but the disease has resisted simple explanations and easy solutions.

One of the main reasons Alzheimer's remains a puzzle is that it doesn't present uniformly. Two individuals with nearly identical brain scans can exhibit vastly different symptoms. Some people with significant plaque buildup live cognitively normal lives, while others with minimal visible damage experience profound decline. This variability has confounded scientists and suggested that Alzheimer's is not a one-size-fits-all disease. Instead, it may represent a spectrum of interrelated conditions, each influenced by a unique combination of genetic, environmental, and lifestyle factors.

Moreover, the field has historically been dominated by a single narrative: the amyloid cascade hypothesis. While this theory provided valuable insights, it also narrowed the scope of research for decades. Billions of dollars have been spent on therapies targeting amyloid plaques, yet none have delivered the transformative results we hoped for. This singular focus has led to missed opportunities in exploring alternative pathways, such as inflammation, vascular health, and the gut-brain connection, which are now emerging as critical pieces of the puzzle.

Another layer of complexity lies in the timing of the disease. Alzheimer's often begins silently, with subtle changes in the brain occurring years—sometimes decades—before symptoms appear. By the time memory loss and cognitive decline become noticeable, the disease has already caused significant damage. This long, hidden progression makes early detection and intervention particularly challenging.

Furthermore, the societal and cultural dimensions of Alzheimer's contribute to its mystique. There is a stigma surrounding cognitive decline that discourages open discussions and delays diagnosis. Many people view memory loss as an inevitable part of aging, ignoring early warning signs until it is too late. This hesitation to address the disease has slowed both public awareness and funding for research.

Yet, despite these challenges, progress is being made. Recent advancements in imaging technology, biomarker identification, and genetic research are shedding new light on the disease. Interdisciplinary approaches are beginning to reveal connections between Alzheimer's and systemic factors like metabolic health and immune function. And perhaps most importantly, the narrative around Alzheimer's is shifting—from one of despair to one of hope.

This book explores the many facets of why Alzheimer's has remained a mystery for so long, but it also seeks to demonstrate how those mysteries are finally being unraveled. By stepping back and looking at the disease through a broader lens, we are discovering new pathways to understanding, treating, and ultimately preventing it.

Alzheimer's may have resisted simple explanations, but as history has shown us, even the most complex puzzles can be solved with the right tools, perspectives, and persistence. As we dive deeper into this book, we'll explore the breakthroughs and insights that are bringing clarity to the shadows and guiding us toward a future where this devastating disease is no longer a mystery—but a memory of the past.

The Stakes: Humanity's Greatest Cognitive Challenge

Alzheimer's disease is not just a medical condition; it is one of the most profound challenges humanity faces in the modern era. At its heart lies a confrontation with something deeply personal: the loss of memory, identity, and connection. This is what makes Alzheimer's uniquely devastating—not only for those who live with it but for the families, caregivers, and communities that support them.

The numbers alone paint a sobering picture. Worldwide, more than 55 million people are living with dementia, a number expected to double every two decades as populations age. In the United States alone, Alzheimer's disease is the sixth leading cause of death, with over 6 million people currently diagnosed. The economic toll is staggering, with the global cost of dementia reaching over $1 trillion annually, a figure that continues to rise. Yet these figures cannot fully capture the emotional cost of watching a loved one slip away, one memory at a time.

But the stakes are far greater than individual lives. Alzheimer's represents a broader challenge to how we understand and treat diseases of the brain. While we've made remarkable strides in curing or managing many physical illnesses, the brain remains a frontier we've only begun to explore. Its intricate networks and astonishing plasticity have made it both fascinating and frustrating for scientists. Unlike a broken bone or clogged artery, the brain's dysfunction is far more complex, involving countless interdependent systems that must work in harmony to sustain cognition, emotion, and personality.

This challenge is exacerbated by the silent, insidious nature of Alzheimer's. The disease begins its work in the brain decades before symptoms appear, making early intervention and prevention strategies particularly difficult to implement. It demands that we rethink how we approach diagnosis, shifting from reactive treatment to proactive detection and care.

Alzheimer's is also a stark reminder of the vulnerabilities that come with aging. As life expectancy increases across the globe, the prevalence of age-related diseases like Alzheimer's will inevitably rise. Without effective treatments, we face a future where more people will live longer lives, but with diminished quality—straining healthcare systems, economies, and families in unprecedented ways.

The stakes go beyond science and medicine; they touch the very fabric of society. Alzheimer's forces us to confront questions about how we value our elders, allocate resources, and build systems of care that prioritize dignity and compassion. It challenges us to ensure that progress in longevity is matched by progress in preserving the quality of those extra years.

Yet, this challenge also presents an extraordinary opportunity. Alzheimer's research is at a tipping point, with breakthroughs in imaging, genetics, and drug development opening doors that were once firmly closed. The growing understanding of systemic factors—such as the role of inflammation, vascular health, and lifestyle—offers hope that this disease is not inevitable. And with that hope comes the possibility of not only curing Alzheimer's but also unlocking new insights into the brain that could revolutionize our understanding of other neurological conditions.

In many ways, the battle against Alzheimer's is about more than this one disease. It is about humanity's capacity to overcome its most daunting challenges through innovation, collaboration, and an unyielding commitment to progress. The stakes are high, but so are the rewards. By addressing Alzheimer's, we are not only preserving memories and relationships but also reaffirming our belief in the resilience of the human spirit.

As we navigate this challenge together, let us remember: the brain is where we live, where we love, and where we dream. Protecting it is not just a medical priority—it is a moral imperative. The fight against Alzheimer's is the fight for our shared humanity, and it is one we cannot afford to lose.

A Breakthrough in Understanding

Every field of science has its watershed moment—a turning point when scattered ideas coalesce into clarity, setting the stage for meaningful progress. For Alzheimer's disease, that moment has arrived. Decades of research, once fragmented and hyper-focused on isolated aspects of the disease, are now converging to reveal a more comprehensive understanding of what drives Alzheimer's and how it can be addressed.

For years, the dominant narrative around Alzheimer's centered on amyloid plaques and tau tangles, the hallmark pathological features identified in the brains of those with the disease. While these discoveries were critical milestones, they failed to fully explain the disease's variability, progression, and resistance to treatment. Now, researchers are recognizing that Alzheimer's is not solely a problem of plaques and tangles but a multi-faceted disorder influenced by a complex interplay of systemic factors.

The breakthrough lies in a paradigm shift—a move from treating Alzheimer's as a singular brain disease to understanding it as a systemic condition with roots in inflammation, metabolism, and even the gut-brain connection. This broader perspective has allowed researchers to ask new questions: How do chronic inflammation and immune system dysfunction accelerate cognitive decline? Why do metabolic conditions like diabetes increase the risk of Alzheimer's? And how do lifestyle factors like diet, exercise, and social engagement play a protective role?

One of the most transformative insights has been the identification of Alzheimer's as a process that begins long before symptoms appear. The early stages of the disease—when brain cells are silently struggling—represent a critical window of opportunity. Armed with advanced imaging techniques and biomarker analysis, scientists can now detect these changes years, even decades, before noticeable cognitive decline. This ability to intervene early is a game-changer, shifting the focus from managing symptoms to preventing the disease altogether.

Another key development is the rise of precision medicine in Alzheimer's care. No two individuals experience Alzheimer's in exactly the same way, and researchers are now uncovering the genetic, environmental, and lifestyle factors that contribute to this variability. With tools like genomics and artificial intelligence, we are entering an era where treatments can be tailored to the unique biology of each patient. This personalized approach holds the promise of greater effectiveness and fewer side effects, paving the way for therapies that truly transform lives.

Breakthroughs in treatment are also emerging, thanks to innovative strategies that target not only the brain but the entire body. Anti-inflammatory drugs, lifestyle interventions, and even dietary changes are showing promise in reducing risk and slowing progression. Novel therapies that promote neurogenesis—the brain's ability to regenerate and repair—are also on the horizon, offering hope for restoring lost cognitive function.

But perhaps the most profound breakthrough is in our collective mindset. The scientific community is moving beyond the idea that Alzheimer's is an inevitable part of aging. We now understand that while age is the greatest risk factor, Alzheimer's is not a natural consequence of growing older. It is a disease—a condition that can be studied, treated, and one day, cured. This shift in perception is inspiring new investments, collaborations, and public awareness campaigns that are accelerating progress.

The journey to understanding Alzheimer's has been long and fraught with challenges, but the breakthroughs of recent years represent a turning point. For the first time, we are seeing a clear path forward—one that blends cutting-edge science with practical interventions and a commitment to early detection and prevention.

This book is rooted in the hope and promise of these discoveries. It aims to translate the complexity of this disease into actionable insights, empowering readers with the knowledge needed to protect themselves and their loved ones. A breakthrough in understanding is only meaningful if it leads to a breakthrough in action, and that is precisely what this moment demands.

We stand on the precipice of change. The pieces of the puzzle are coming together, and with each new discovery, we are closer to unraveling Alzheimer's once and for all.

Part I: The Origins of Alzheimer's Disease

Chapter 1: The History of Alzheimer's

From Alois Alzheimer to Modern Research

The story of Alzheimer's disease begins over a century ago, in 1906, when a German psychiatrist and neurologist named Alois Alzheimer presented his groundbreaking findings at a medical conference in Tübingen, Germany. He described the case of a 51-year-old woman named Auguste Deter, who had been admitted to the hospital with severe memory loss, confusion, and unpredictable behavior. After her death, Dr. Alzheimer conducted a post-mortem examination of her brain and discovered two abnormalities that would define the disease: unusual protein deposits, later called amyloid plaques, and tangled fibers inside neurons, now known as neurofibrillary tangles.

At the time, these findings were a scientific curiosity, and Alzheimer's work went largely unnoticed. In fact, it wasn't until the 1910s that Emil Kraepelin, a prominent psychiatrist and Alzheimer's mentor, named the condition "Alzheimer's disease" in his influential textbook. For decades, the disease was thought to be rare, affecting only younger patients in what was termed "presenile dementia." It wasn't until the mid-20th century that researchers began to recognize its broader prevalence among older adults and its distinction from general senility.

The advent of advanced microscopic techniques in the 1960s reignited interest in Alzheimer's pathology. Scientists began to focus on amyloid plaques and tau tangles, which had been overlooked for decades. These discoveries set the stage for the amyloid cascade hypothesis, proposed in the 1990s, which posited that the accumulation of amyloid-beta protein was the central driver of the disease. This theory dominated Alzheimer's research for years, shaping the development of diagnostic tools and potential treatments.

In parallel, genetic research made significant strides in the late 20th century. In 1991, mutations in the amyloid precursor protein (APP) gene were linked to familial Alzheimer's disease, a rare but devastating inherited form of the condition. This discovery, followed by the identification of mutations in the presenilin 1 and 2 genes, cemented the idea that genetics played a crucial role in certain cases of Alzheimer's. Yet, for the vast majority of patients with sporadic Alzheimer's, the causes remained elusive.

The introduction of neuroimaging technologies in the late 20th century provided researchers with new tools to observe Alzheimer's in living patients. Techniques like PET scans and MRI allowed for the visualization of brain atrophy and amyloid deposition, offering unprecedented insights into the disease's progression. These advancements spurred an era of rapid growth in Alzheimer's research, bringing both promise and frustration.

While many strides were made, the 21st century brought a sobering realization: decades of effort to develop amyloid-targeting therapies had not yielded the hoped-for results. Clinical trials consistently failed to show meaningful improvements in symptoms or disease progression, raising questions about the amyloid cascade hypothesis and prompting researchers to look beyond plaques and tangles.

Today, Alzheimer's research stands at a crossroads. The field has expanded to explore a wide array of contributing factors, from chronic inflammation and vascular health to the microbiome and lifestyle influences. Scientists now recognize that Alzheimer's is not a singular disease but a complex interplay of genetic, environmental, and systemic factors that vary from person to person.

This broader understanding has given rise to interdisciplinary approaches and collaborative efforts that bring together experts in neurology, immunology, and metabolic health. The work of Dr. Alzheimer laid the foundation, but the modern pursuit of answers has transformed the field into a global endeavor, driven by the hope that uncovering the origins of this disease will unlock the path to prevention and cure.

The journey from Dr. Alzheimer's first observations to today's research highlights both the incredible progress we've made and the challenges that lie ahead. Understanding the history of Alzheimer's is essential for appreciating how far we've come—and how much further we must go to unravel its mysteries and transform the lives of millions.

Missteps and Breakthroughs Over the Decades

The history of Alzheimer's disease is one of both remarkable breakthroughs and frustrating missteps, a reflection of the complexity of this condition and the challenges inherent in understanding it. While scientific advances have brought us closer to unraveling Alzheimer's, some paths, once thought promising, have proven to be dead ends, and certain assumptions have hindered progress.

In the early 20th century, shortly after Alois Alzheimer's initial discovery, the disease largely faded into obscurity. For decades, it was viewed as a rare disorder affecting only younger individuals, relegated to the fringes of medical research. This misconception delayed widespread recognition of Alzheimer's as a major public health issue and stalled efforts to study its broader implications. The condition was often dismissed as "senility," an unavoidable consequence of aging, rather than a distinct pathological process.

It wasn't until the mid-20th century that researchers began to see Alzheimer's for what it was: a disease with identifiable patterns and distinct neuropathological features. However, this period was marked by significant oversights. Early research fixated on describing the visible hallmarks of the disease—amyloid plaques and tau tangles—without fully investigating the underlying mechanisms. The tools and technologies of the time limited deeper exploration, and much of the field's energy went into cataloging rather than understanding.

The introduction of the amyloid cascade hypothesis in the 1990s was both a breakthrough and a bottleneck. The hypothesis proposed that the accumulation of amyloid-beta protein was the central trigger for Alzheimer's, with downstream effects, including tau tangles and neuronal death. Initially, this theory sparked hope. It provided a clear target for drug development, and researchers believed they were on the verge of a cure.

However, the decades that followed revealed the limitations of this approach. Billions of dollars were invested in amyloid-targeting therapies, yet clinical trial after clinical trial failed to produce meaningful improvements in symptoms or disease progression. These failures underscored a critical misstep: the field had become overly reliant on a single narrative. By focusing so intently on amyloid, researchers overlooked other potentially significant contributors, such as inflammation, vascular health, and the immune system's role in brain function.

Another challenge was the inability to detect Alzheimer's in its earliest stages. For much of the 20th century, the disease could only be definitively diagnosed post-mortem, leaving researchers with an incomplete understanding of its progression. This limitation meant that many studies focused on patients in the later stages of the disease, missing opportunities to explore its origins or intervene earlier.

Despite these setbacks, there have been significant breakthroughs that have reshaped the field. Advances in neuroimaging and biomarker detection have revolutionized how Alzheimer's is studied and diagnosed. Tools like PET scans and cerebrospinal fluid analysis now allow researchers to observe amyloid buildup and tau tangles in living patients, paving the way for earlier detection and more targeted interventions.

Genetic research has also yielded important insights. The identification of the APOE4 gene as a major risk factor for Alzheimer's, along with discoveries about familial mutations in the

APP, presenilin 1, and presenilin 2 genes, has deepened our understanding of the disease's hereditary aspects. These findings have not only clarified the genetic underpinnings of Alzheimer's but also opened doors to exploring epigenetics and how lifestyle and environment can influence gene expression.

Perhaps the most profound breakthrough has been the realization that Alzheimer's is not solely a neurological disease but a systemic one, influenced by factors such as inflammation, metabolic health, and even the microbiome. This shift in understanding has sparked new lines of inquiry and interdisciplinary collaborations, moving the field away from a narrow focus on amyloid and toward a more holistic approach.

The history of Alzheimer's research is a testament to both the power and the pitfalls of scientific discovery. Each breakthrough has brought us closer to understanding the disease, while each misstep has provided valuable lessons about the importance of keeping an open mind and exploring multiple avenues. As we look back on the journey, it becomes clear that progress is rarely linear. Yet, with every failure, the scientific community has grown more resilient and better equipped to tackle one of humanity's greatest challenges.

The road to unraveling Alzheimer's has been long and winding, but it is this very history—of persistence, curiosity, and adaptation—that gives us hope for the future. Each misstep has ultimately contributed to the breakthroughs that will one day lead to a world free from this devastating disease.

Chapter 2: The Biology of Memory and Brain Aging

Understanding the Healthy Brain

To understand Alzheimer's disease and its devastating effects, we must first appreciate the intricate workings of a healthy brain. The brain is the most complex organ in the human body, a three-pound marvel that serves as the command center for every thought, emotion, and action. It is a dynamic and adaptive network, capable of remarkable feats of learning, memory, and problem-solving.

At its core, the brain is composed of approximately 86 billion neurons, specialized cells that transmit information through electrical and chemical signals. These neurons form vast, interconnected networks that enable communication between different regions of the brain. Each neuron connects to thousands of others through synapses, creating a web of activity that underlies everything from basic motor functions to higher-order cognition.

Memory, a key function of the brain, relies on these neuronal networks. The hippocampus, a seahorse-shaped structure in the brain's medial temporal lobe, plays a central role in forming and retrieving memories. It acts as a sort of "gateway," processing and organizing new information before passing it along to other regions for long-term storage. Meanwhile, the prefrontal cortex, located at the front of the brain, manages working memory and decision-making, ensuring that we can hold information in mind and use it to guide our actions.

The brain's ability to adapt and reorganize itself—a phenomenon known as neuroplasticity—is essential for learning and memory. When we learn something new, synapses strengthen or weaken, forming new pathways or refining existing ones. This adaptability is why the brain can recover from injuries, build new skills, and retain knowledge throughout life.

However, the brain's efficiency depends on more than just its neurons. Glial cells, often referred to as the brain's support system, play critical roles in maintaining neuronal health. Astrocytes provide nutrients and regulate the chemical environment, while microglia act as the brain's immune cells, clearing away debris and responding to injury or infection. Oligodendrocytes produce myelin, the insulating sheath that allows for the rapid transmission of electrical signals along neurons. Together, these cells ensure that the brain operates smoothly and effectively.

Another key aspect of a healthy brain is its ability to clear waste. During sleep, the glymphatic system—a network of channels in the brain—flushes out toxins, including proteins like amyloid-beta. This process is vital for preventing the accumulation of harmful substances that could interfere with neuronal function.

Despite its remarkable capabilities, the brain is not invincible. Over time, it undergoes natural changes associated with aging. These changes include reduced synaptic density, slower signal transmission, and a gradual decline in the efficiency of the glymphatic system. While these processes are a normal part of aging, they can make the brain more vulnerable to diseases like Alzheimer's.

One of the most important factors in maintaining a healthy brain is its connection to the rest of the body. The brain does not function in isolation; it relies on a steady supply of oxygen and nutrients delivered through the vascular system. The blood-brain barrier, a protective filter, ensures that harmful substances do not enter the brain while allowing essential nutrients to pass through. However, disruptions to this barrier or impairments in blood flow can have profound effects on brain health, highlighting the importance of cardiovascular health in preventing cognitive decline.

In a healthy brain, all these systems work in harmony to support memory, learning, and overall cognitive function. This intricate balance allows us to experience the richness of life, form meaningful connections, and navigate the world with clarity and purpose.

Understanding the healthy brain is not just an academic exercise; it provides the foundation for identifying what goes wrong in Alzheimer's disease. By examining the normal processes of memory formation, neural communication, and waste clearance, we gain critical insights into how these systems break down and how they might be restored. The healthy brain is not just a marvel of biology—it is the standard against which we measure the damage caused by Alzheimer's and the goal toward which every treatment and prevention strategy aspires.

How Aging Impacts Neurological Function

Aging is an inevitable process, and its effects on the brain are both profound and multifaceted. While the brain demonstrates remarkable adaptability and resilience throughout life, aging introduces subtle changes that can gradually affect its structure and function. These changes, while normal, set the stage for vulnerabilities that may contribute to conditions like Alzheimer's disease if compounded by other factors.

One of the most noticeable effects of aging on the brain is a reduction in brain volume, a process known as atrophy. This shrinkage primarily affects areas critical for memory and cognition, such as the hippocampus and prefrontal cortex. Although some degree of atrophy is a natural part of aging, excessive loss of brain tissue can impair cognitive abilities and increase the risk of neurodegenerative diseases.

Another hallmark of aging is the decline in synaptic density, the intricate network of connections between neurons. As we age, the number and strength of these synapses can diminish, leading to slower information processing and reduced plasticity—the brain's ability to adapt and form new pathways. This decline is a key factor in the gradual slowing of cognitive functions, such as learning new skills or recalling detailed information.

The efficiency of neuronal communication also decreases with age. This is partly due to changes in the production and availability of neurotransmitters, the chemical messengers that facilitate communication between neurons. For instance, dopamine levels tend to decline with age, impacting functions like motivation and reward processing. Similarly, reductions in acetylcholine, a neurotransmitter essential for memory and attention, can impair cognitive performance.

The aging brain also faces challenges in maintaining its internal maintenance and repair systems. One critical process affected by aging is the brain's ability to clear waste products, including amyloid-beta, a protein associated with Alzheimer's disease. During sleep, the glymphatic system facilitates the removal of these proteins, but with age, this system becomes less efficient. Over time, the accumulation of amyloid-beta and other toxins can interfere with normal neuronal function and increase the risk of neurodegenerative conditions.

Inflammation, a natural response to injury or infection, also plays a complex role in the aging brain. In younger individuals, the brain's immune cells, particularly microglia, work effectively to protect neurons and clear debris. However, as the brain ages, these cells can become overactive or dysfunctional, leading to chronic low-level inflammation. This state, often referred to as "inflammaging," has been implicated in the progression of cognitive decline and neurodegenerative diseases.

Another critical aspect of aging is the decline in the vascular health of the brain. The brain relies on a consistent and robust blood supply to deliver oxygen and nutrients while removing waste products. With age, blood vessels may stiffen or narrow, reducing blood flow to the brain. Additionally, the blood-brain barrier, which protects the brain from harmful substances, can become more permeable, increasing the risk of damage from toxins or pathogens. These vascular changes can significantly impact cognitive function and increase the risk of developing conditions like Alzheimer's.

Despite these challenges, it is important to recognize that aging does not necessarily equate to cognitive decline. Many individuals maintain sharp cognitive abilities well into old age, demonstrating the remarkable variability in how aging impacts neurological function. Factors such as genetics, lifestyle, and environmental influences play crucial roles in determining the extent to which aging affects the brain.

Exercise, a healthy diet, intellectual engagement, and social connections have all been shown to promote brain health and mitigate the effects of aging. These factors support neurogenesis (the growth of new neurons), enhance synaptic plasticity, and improve vascular health, providing a buffer against age-related decline.

Understanding how aging impacts neurological function is essential for identifying the early signs of pathological changes, such as those seen in Alzheimer's disease. By distinguishing between normal aging and the early stages of neurodegeneration, researchers and clinicians can develop targeted interventions to preserve cognitive health and improve quality of life for aging populations. Aging may bring challenges, but it also offers opportunities for proactive strategies to protect and nurture the brain throughout life.

Chapter 3: Plaques, Tangles, and Beyond

The Amyloid Cascade Hypothesis

For decades, the amyloid cascade hypothesis has been the cornerstone of Alzheimer's research. Proposed in the early 1990s, this theory centers on the idea that the accumulation of amyloid-beta protein in the brain is the primary driver of Alzheimer's disease, triggering a series of pathological events that ultimately lead to cognitive decline. While the hypothesis has been instrumental in advancing our understanding of Alzheimer's, it has also sparked significant debate, highlighting both its strengths and its limitations.

The hypothesis begins with the production of amyloid-beta, a protein fragment derived from the cleavage of a larger protein called amyloid precursor protein (APP). In healthy brains, amyloid-beta is typically cleared away efficiently. However, in Alzheimer's, this balance is disrupted, leading to the accumulation of amyloid-beta into sticky plaques that deposit between neurons. These plaques are considered the first step in a cascade of events that include the formation of tau tangles, inflammation, neuronal dysfunction, and, ultimately, brain cell death.

Support for the amyloid cascade hypothesis emerged from several key discoveries. Mutations in genes related to APP and presenilin proteins, which are involved in amyloid-beta production, were found to cause rare familial forms of Alzheimer's. These genetic links reinforced the idea that amyloid-beta plays a central role in the disease process. Additionally, amyloid plaques were identified as a defining pathological feature of Alzheimer's, observed consistently in post-mortem brain studies.

The hypothesis also provided a clear target for drug development. Over the past two decades, significant resources have been devoted to creating therapies aimed at reducing amyloid-beta levels in the brain. These efforts have included drugs that inhibit its production, promote its clearance, or prevent it from aggregating into plaques.

Despite its influence, the amyloid cascade hypothesis has faced considerable challenges. Most notably, clinical trials targeting amyloid-beta have largely failed to produce meaningful improvements in cognitive outcomes. While some treatments successfully reduced amyloid levels, they did not halt or reverse the progression of Alzheimer's. This disconnect between amyloid reduction and clinical benefit has raised questions about whether amyloid-beta is the root cause of Alzheimer's or merely a byproduct of the disease process.

Moreover, some individuals with significant amyloid plaque buildup in their brains show no signs of cognitive impairment, while others with minimal plaques experience severe symptoms. This variability suggests that amyloid may be one piece of a larger puzzle rather than the sole driver of the disease.

Critics of the hypothesis argue that the field's intense focus on amyloid-beta has overshadowed other important contributors to Alzheimer's, such as inflammation, vascular dysfunction, and metabolic disturbances. Emerging research highlights the complex interplay between these factors, suggesting that Alzheimer's is not a linear cascade but a multifaceted condition with multiple pathways leading to cognitive decline.

Nonetheless, the amyloid cascade hypothesis remains a foundational framework for understanding Alzheimer's. It has driven significant advances in our knowledge of the disease and continues to inform ongoing research. Recent developments, such as the approval of amyloid-targeting drugs that may offer modest benefits for certain patients, indicate that amyloid-beta still plays a role, even if it is not the whole story.

The evolving perspective on the amyloid cascade hypothesis underscores the importance of adopting a broader, more integrative approach to Alzheimer's research. While amyloid-beta remains a critical piece of the puzzle, the future of Alzheimer's science lies in understanding how this protein interacts with other factors to drive the disease. By expanding our focus beyond plaques and tangles, we can uncover new pathways to prevention and treatment, moving closer to unraveling the full complexity of Alzheimer's.

Tau Tangles: A Closer Look

While amyloid plaques have often dominated the spotlight in Alzheimer's research, tau tangles are an equally critical feature of the disease, offering another lens through which to understand its progression. Unlike plaques, which form between neurons, tau tangles occur inside the neurons themselves, disrupting their structural integrity and function. Understanding tau's role in Alzheimer's has become a key focus of modern research, revealing insights into how these tangles contribute to cognitive decline.

Tau is a protein found within neurons, where it plays a vital role in stabilizing microtubules—structures that act as the cell's transport system. Microtubules are essential for moving nutrients, molecules, and waste products to and from the neuron's cell body and its extensions, such as axons and dendrites. In a healthy brain, tau binds to microtubules in a carefully regulated manner, ensuring the efficient operation of this intracellular transport system.

However, in Alzheimer's disease, tau becomes abnormally hyperphosphorylated—a chemical modification that causes tau to detach from microtubules and clump together. These clumps form twisted, insoluble fibers known as neurofibrillary tangles, which accumulate within neurons. As tangles spread, they destabilize the microtubules, disrupting the neuron's ability to transport essential materials and leading to cellular dysfunction and, eventually, cell death.

The presence of tau tangles correlates more closely with cognitive decline than amyloid plaques, suggesting that tau pathology plays a central role in driving the symptoms of Alzheimer's. Research has shown that the spread of tau tangles follows a characteristic pattern, starting in the entorhinal cortex and hippocampus—regions critical for memory and learning—before advancing to other areas of the brain. This progression aligns with the typical trajectory of Alzheimer's symptoms, which often begin with memory loss and later affect executive functions, language, and spatial awareness.

One of the most intriguing aspects of tau pathology is its apparent ability to propagate from one neuron to another. Studies suggest that misfolded tau can spread along connected networks of neurons, acting almost like a "prion," or infectious protein. This discovery has profound implications for understanding how Alzheimer's progresses and offers a potential target for interventions aimed at halting the spread of tau tangles.

Despite its importance, the exact triggers for tau dysfunction remain unclear. While amyloid plaques have been hypothesized to initiate tau pathology in Alzheimer's, this relationship is not fully understood. Tau tangles are also found in other neurodegenerative diseases, such as frontotemporal dementia and chronic traumatic encephalopathy, indicating that tau dysfunction is not exclusive to Alzheimer's. This broader context highlights the complexity of tau's role and suggests that it may act as a final common pathway in various forms of neuronal degeneration.

Efforts to develop tau-targeting therapies have gained momentum in recent years. Experimental treatments include compounds designed to prevent tau phosphorylation, promote the clearance of abnormal tau, or block its spread between neurons. Early results from clinical trials are promising, offering hope that these approaches could complement existing therapies focused on amyloid-beta.

The study of tau tangles has also shed light on the brain's vulnerability to stressors, such as inflammation and oxidative damage. These factors can exacerbate tau pathology, underscoring the importance of a holistic approach to treating Alzheimer's that addresses the broader environment in which these pathologies develop.

Tau tangles represent a critical piece of the Alzheimer's puzzle, linking the molecular changes within neurons to the functional impairments observed in patients. By unraveling the mechanisms behind tau dysfunction, researchers are opening new avenues for understanding the disease and developing targeted therapies. While amyloid plaques may initiate the cascade of events, it is tau tangles that may hold the key to halting the disease's relentless progression. As science delves deeper into the intricacies of tau, it brings us closer to unlocking solutions that can preserve the delicate balance of the brain's intricate machinery.

Revisiting the Role of Neuroinflammation

For many years, the focus of Alzheimer's research remained squarely on amyloid plaques and tau tangles. However, mounting evidence has highlighted the critical role of neuroinflammation in the disease process. Far from being a secondary effect of plaque and tangle formation, inflammation is now recognized as a central driver of Alzheimer's pathology, shaping the progression and severity of the disease.

Neuroinflammation is the brain's immune response to threats such as injury, infection, or the accumulation of abnormal proteins like amyloid-beta. In healthy circumstances, this response is beneficial. Microglia, the brain's primary immune cells, act as sentinels, clearing debris, damaged neurons, and toxic substances. Astrocytes, another type of glial cell, help maintain the brain's chemical balance and provide support to neurons. Together, these cells form a critical defense system that preserves brain function.

In Alzheimer's, however, this immune response becomes dysregulated. Amyloid plaques and tau tangles trigger microglia to activate, releasing inflammatory molecules such as cytokines and chemokines. While initially protective, chronic activation of microglia leads to a sustained inflammatory state that damages surrounding neurons and exacerbates the spread of tau tangles. Similarly, astrocytes can shift from their supportive role to a reactive state, further amplifying the inflammatory environment.

One of the most intriguing aspects of neuroinflammation is its bidirectional relationship with Alzheimer's pathology. While plaques and tangles can initiate inflammation, the inflammatory response itself accelerates the accumulation of these pathological features. For example, chronic inflammation can impair the glymphatic system, the brain's waste clearance mechanism, reducing the removal of amyloid-beta. This feedback loop creates a vicious cycle in which inflammation and Alzheimer's pathology fuel each other.

Genetic studies have provided additional support for the role of neuroinflammation in Alzheimer's. Variants in genes such as TREM2, which affects microglial function, have been linked to an increased risk of the disease. These findings underscore the importance of the immune system in Alzheimer's and suggest that targeting inflammation could be a viable therapeutic strategy.

Moreover, neuroinflammation is not an isolated phenomenon but is influenced by systemic factors. Chronic conditions such as diabetes, cardiovascular disease, and obesity are associated with low-grade inflammation that can cross the blood-brain barrier and exacerbate neuroinflammatory processes. Similarly, infections, stress, and poor sleep can heighten systemic inflammation, potentially contributing to the development or progression of Alzheimer's.

Despite its importance, neuroinflammation remains a challenging target for treatment. The brain's immune system is highly complex, and suppressing inflammation indiscriminately could interfere with its protective functions. Current research is focused on finding ways to modulate, rather than completely inhibit, the inflammatory response. This includes identifying drugs that can shift microglia and astrocytes back to their protective states or block specific inflammatory pathways without disrupting overall immune activity.

Lifestyle interventions also play a role in managing neuroinflammation. Regular exercise, a healthy diet rich in anti-inflammatory compounds, stress reduction, and quality sleep have all been shown to reduce systemic inflammation and promote brain health. These approaches may not only slow the progression of Alzheimer's but also help prevent it from developing in the first place.

Revisiting the role of neuroinflammation has fundamentally

changed the way researchers and clinicians view Alzheimer's. It is no longer seen merely as a disease of protein misfolding but as a dynamic interaction between the brain's immune system and its environment. By addressing neuroinflammation, we open new doors to treatments that could break the cycle of damage and bring us closer to halting the disease's progression.

As Alzheimer's research continues to evolve, understanding and targeting neuroinflammation will remain a critical piece of the puzzle. This deeper appreciation of the brain's immune system not only enhances our grasp of Alzheimer's but also holds promise for treating a range of neurodegenerative diseases. By restoring balance to this vital system, we move one step closer to preserving the brain's function and resilience against the challenges of aging and disease.

Chapter 4: The Missing Puzzle Piece

The Role of Mitochondrial Dysfunction

Among the emerging areas of Alzheimer's research, mitochondrial dysfunction stands out as a critical but often overlooked factor in the disease's progression. Mitochondria, often referred to as the "powerhouses" of the cell, are essential for producing the energy that neurons require to function. Unlike many other cell types, neurons rely almost entirely on mitochondrial energy to support their high metabolic demands, making them particularly vulnerable to mitochondrial dysfunction.

In the healthy brain, mitochondria provide a steady supply of adenosine triphosphate (ATP), the molecule that powers cellular processes. They also regulate calcium levels, produce key signaling molecules, and help protect cells from oxidative stress by neutralizing harmful reactive oxygen species (ROS). However, in Alzheimer's disease, these functions become impaired, leading to energy deficits, oxidative damage, and neuronal dysfunction.

One of the earliest signs of mitochondrial dysfunction in Alzheimer's is a reduction in mitochondrial efficiency. This means that mitochondria produce less ATP while generating more ROS, which can damage cellular components such as DNA, proteins, and lipids. This oxidative stress is particularly damaging in the brain, where the high lipid content of neuronal membranes makes them highly susceptible to ROS-induced damage.

Mitochondrial dysfunction also disrupts calcium homeostasis, another key aspect of neuronal health. Mitochondria play a vital role in buffering calcium levels within cells, preventing toxic buildup. When this regulation fails, excess calcium can trigger cell death pathways, further contributing to neuronal loss in Alzheimer's.

The connection between mitochondrial dysfunction and Alzheimer's pathology extends to amyloid-beta and tau, the hallmark features of the disease. Studies have shown that amyloid-beta can directly impair mitochondrial function by embedding in mitochondrial membranes, disrupting their structure and function. Similarly, abnormal tau can interfere with the transport of mitochondria along axons and dendrites, cutting off the supply of energy to critical parts of the neuron. This creates a vicious cycle in which mitochondrial dysfunction exacerbates amyloid and tau pathology, and vice versa.

Genetic evidence further supports the role of mitochondria in Alzheimer's. Variants in genes involved in mitochondrial function, such as those regulating oxidative phosphorylation, have been associated with an increased risk of the disease. Additionally, mitochondria possess their own DNA, separate from the cell's nuclear DNA, and mutations in mitochondrial DNA accumulate with age. These mutations can impair mitochondrial function, contributing to the age-related decline in brain health that increases susceptibility to Alzheimer's.

Mitochondrial dysfunction also links Alzheimer's to systemic factors such as metabolic health. Conditions like diabetes and obesity, which impair mitochondrial function in the body, are well-established risk factors for Alzheimer's. Insulin resistance, in particular, affects mitochondrial efficiency and exacerbates oxidative stress, highlighting the interconnected nature of brain and systemic health.

Efforts to address mitochondrial dysfunction in Alzheimer's are gaining momentum. Experimental therapies aim to enhance mitochondrial function, reduce oxidative stress, or prevent amyloid-beta and tau from interfering with mitochondrial processes. Strategies such as boosting mitochondrial biogenesis (the creation of new mitochondria) and improving mitochondrial dynamics (the balance between fusion and fission) show promise in preclinical studies.

Lifestyle interventions that support mitochondrial health are also being explored. Regular exercise, for example, has been shown to improve mitochondrial efficiency and reduce oxidative stress in the brain. A diet rich in antioxidants, along with strategies like intermittent fasting or a ketogenic diet, may also enhance mitochondrial function and resilience.

The role of mitochondrial dysfunction in Alzheimer's highlights the need for a broader understanding of the disease beyond plaques and tangles. Mitochondria sit at the intersection of energy production, oxidative stress, and cell signaling, making them a central player in the health of neurons. By targeting this critical component of cellular function, we may uncover new ways to halt or even reverse the progression of Alzheimer's.

As research into mitochondrial dysfunction continues to evolve, it offers a powerful reminder that Alzheimer's is a multifaceted disease requiring a multifaceted approach. Addressing this "missing puzzle piece" may not only provide new therapeutic targets but also deepen our understanding of how the brain's energy systems sustain cognition and resilience throughout life.

Environmental Triggers and Lifestyle Factors

Alzheimer's disease has long been understood as a complex interplay of genetic predisposition, biological processes, and environmental influences. While much research has focused on the internal mechanisms of the disease—such as plaques, tangles, and inflammation—emerging evidence highlights the profound impact of environmental triggers and lifestyle factors. These external influences not only shape the risk of developing Alzheimer's but may also determine the timing and severity of its progression.

The Environmental Connection

Environmental factors encompass a wide range of exposures, from air pollution and toxins to dietary habits and social engagement. Among these, air pollution has garnered increasing attention for its role in neurodegenerative diseases. Tiny particles known as particulate matter (PM2.5) can enter the bloodstream and cross the blood-brain barrier, triggering inflammation and oxidative stress in the brain. Studies have shown that individuals exposed to high levels of air pollution over time are at a significantly greater risk of developing dementia, including Alzheimer's.

Similarly, exposure to heavy metals such as lead, mercury, and cadmium has been linked to cognitive decline. These toxins can accumulate in the brain, disrupting neural processes and exacerbating oxidative damage. Even low-level exposure to these substances, particularly during critical periods of development or aging, may have long-term consequences for brain health.

Sleep quality is another critical environmental factor. Sleep is essential for the brain's glymphatic system, which clears toxins like amyloid-beta. Chronic sleep deprivation or conditions such as sleep apnea can impair this process, leading to a buildup of harmful proteins and an increased risk of Alzheimer's.

The Role of Lifestyle

Lifestyle choices are among the most modifiable factors influencing Alzheimer's risk. Diet, exercise, social engagement, and mental stimulation all play significant roles in shaping brain health. A diet rich in whole foods, particularly those found in the Mediterranean or MIND (Mediterranean-DASH Intervention for Neurodegenerative Delay) diets, has been associated with a lower risk of Alzheimer's. These diets emphasize fruits, vegetables, whole grains, healthy fats, and lean proteins while minimizing processed foods and added sugars. The antioxidants and anti-inflammatory compounds in these foods help protect neurons from damage and support overall brain health.

Physical activity is another powerful protective factor. Regular aerobic exercise improves cardiovascular health, increases blood flow to the brain, and promotes the release of brain-derived neurotrophic factor (BDNF), a protein that supports the growth and survival of neurons. Exercise has also been shown to reduce systemic inflammation and improve insulin sensitivity, both of which are critical for maintaining cognitive function.

Social and mental engagement can also act as buffers against

Alzheimer's. Maintaining strong social connections and engaging in intellectually stimulating activities, such as learning new skills, solving puzzles, or reading, helps build cognitive reserve—the brain's ability to adapt and compensate for damage. A rich social and intellectual life is associated with delayed onset of Alzheimer's symptoms, even in individuals with significant brain pathology.

Stress and Brain Health

Chronic stress has emerged as a significant risk factor for Alzheimer's. Prolonged activation of the body's stress response can lead to elevated levels of cortisol, a hormone that, in excess, can damage the hippocampus, the brain region responsible for memory. Stress can also exacerbate inflammation and impair the brain's ability to repair itself. Practices such as mindfulness, meditation, and stress management techniques have shown promise in mitigating these effects and promoting brain resilience.

A Holistic Perspective

The influence of environmental triggers and lifestyle factors underscores the importance of a holistic approach to Alzheimer's prevention and management. While genetic predisposition cannot be changed, the way individuals interact with their environment and care for their bodies plays a critical role in shaping their risk. The interplay between these factors is complex, with some triggers amplifying or mitigating others. For example, a healthy diet and regular exercise can counteract some of the effects of poor air quality or chronic stress.

Recognizing the role of environmental and lifestyle factors also shifts the narrative around Alzheimer's from inevitability to empowerment. By addressing these modifiable risk factors, individuals and communities can take proactive steps to reduce their risk and improve their overall quality of life. Public health initiatives aimed at reducing pollution, improving access to healthy foods, and encouraging physical activity could have a profound impact on the prevalence of Alzheimer's and other forms of dementia.

As research continues to uncover the connections between

environment, lifestyle, and Alzheimer's, it becomes increasingly clear that this disease is not merely a product of aging or genetics. By understanding and addressing these external influences, we take another important step toward unraveling the mystery of Alzheimer's and unlocking a future where prevention is not only possible but achievable.

Genetics vs. Epigenetics

The relationship between genetics and Alzheimer's disease has been a key focus of research for decades. While genetic predisposition plays a significant role in determining the risk of developing Alzheimer's, it is becoming increasingly clear that genes alone do not tell the whole story. The emerging field of epigenetics—the study of how environmental and lifestyle factors influence gene expression—offers new insights into the origins of Alzheimer's and how its progression might be influenced or even prevented.

The Genetic Landscape

Genetics has provided a strong foundation for understanding Alzheimer's disease. Mutations in specific genes, such as **APP (amyloid precursor protein)** and **PSEN1/PSEN2 (presenilin 1 and 2)**, are linked to early-onset familial Alzheimer's disease, a rare but devastating form of the condition that accounts for less than 5% of cases. These mutations lead to increased production of amyloid-beta, driving the formation of plaques and triggering the disease at a relatively young age.

For the far more common late-onset Alzheimer's, the genetic risk is more complex. The **APOE (apolipoprotein E)** gene has emerged as a major player. Individuals who inherit one copy of the **APOE4** variant have an increased risk of developing Alzheimer's, while those with two copies face an even greater likelihood. APOE4 is thought to influence the accumulation and clearance of amyloid-beta, as well as the brain's response to inflammation.

However, having a genetic predisposition does not guarantee the development of Alzheimer's. Many individuals with one or even two APOE4 alleles never develop the disease, while some without any known genetic risk factors do. This variability points to the influence of other factors—environmental, lifestyle, and epigenetic—that modulate genetic risk.

The Role of Epigenetics

Epigenetics bridges the gap between genetic predisposition and environmental influence. Unlike genetic mutations, which are fixed, epigenetic changes are reversible modifications to DNA or its associated proteins that affect gene activity without altering the underlying sequence. These changes, which include DNA methylation, histone modification, and non-coding RNA regulation, are influenced by factors such as diet, exercise, stress, and exposure to toxins.

In Alzheimer's disease, epigenetic changes have been observed in genes related to amyloid-beta production, tau processing, inflammation, and synaptic function. For example, excessive methylation of certain genes may silence their expression, impairing processes critical for neuronal health. Conversely, reduced methylation of other genes could lead to overactivation of pathways that promote inflammation or oxidative stress.

Lifestyle and environmental factors play a pivotal role in shaping these epigenetic patterns. A healthy diet rich in nutrients such as folate and omega-3 fatty acids can support DNA methylation and reduce inflammation, while regular exercise has been shown to influence the expression of genes involved in neuroprotection. Chronic stress, on the other hand, can alter epigenetic markers in ways that impair memory and increase vulnerability to neurodegenerative processes.

Gene-Environment Interaction

The interplay between genetics and epigenetics underscores the complexity of Alzheimer's. For example, individuals with the APOE4 variant may be more sensitive to environmental triggers, such as poor diet or air pollution, that exacerbate amyloid-beta accumulation or inflammation. Similarly, those with protective genetic profiles may still develop Alzheimer's if exposed to chronic stress, sedentary lifestyles, or other harmful influences that negatively impact gene expression.

Research into gene-environment interaction is revealing ways to counteract genetic risk through targeted interventions. For instance, while APOE4 carriers are at higher risk, studies suggest that adopting a brain-healthy lifestyle—one that includes regular exercise, cognitive engagement, and a nutrient-dense diet—can significantly reduce the likelihood of developing Alzheimer's, even in genetically predisposed individuals.

Implications for Prevention and Treatment

Understanding the dynamic relationship between genetics and epigenetics opens new doors for Alzheimer's prevention and treatment. Epigenetic modifications are reversible, which means they can be targeted with lifestyle interventions, drugs, or even precision therapies that reset harmful epigenetic patterns.

Emerging therapies include compounds designed to modulate DNA methylation or histone acetylation, as well as approaches to boost the activity of neuroprotective genes. Personalized medicine, which takes into account an individual's genetic and epigenetic profile, holds promise for tailoring interventions that maximize efficacy and minimize risk.

Moving Forward

The distinction between genetics and epigenetics is not a dichotomy but a partnership. Genes provide the blueprint, but epigenetic changes determine how that blueprint is read and executed. This dynamic relationship highlights the potential for individuals to influence their Alzheimer's risk through the choices they make and the environments they inhabit.

As research continues to unravel the complexities of genetics and epigenetics, it brings with it a hopeful message: Alzheimer's is not solely dictated by destiny. By understanding and addressing the factors that shape gene expression, we move closer to empowering individuals to take control of their brain health and unlocking new strategies to prevent and treat this devastating disease.

Chapter 5: Root Cause Revealed

Synthesizing Decades of Evidence

Alzheimer's disease is a complex tapestry woven from many threads: amyloid plaques, tau tangles, inflammation, mitochondrial dysfunction, environmental triggers, and genetic predisposition. For decades, researchers have worked tirelessly to isolate the "root cause" of this devastating condition. Yet, the quest has repeatedly revealed a more intricate story—one that resists simplistic explanations. To truly understand Alzheimer's, we must synthesize decades of evidence and acknowledge its multifactorial nature.

The prevailing theories of Alzheimer's have each provided critical insights. The amyloid cascade hypothesis shined a spotlight on the accumulation of amyloid-beta as a trigger for downstream pathology. The identification of tau tangles connected neuronal dysfunction directly to the loss of cognitive function. Neuroinflammation illuminated the role of the brain's immune response, while mitochondrial dysfunction underscored the importance of energy production and cellular health. Each of these discoveries represents a piece of the puzzle, but no single theory can fully explain the disease's complexity.

A major breakthrough in synthesizing these findings came with the realization that Alzheimer's is not a disease with a single cause but rather the result of a confluence of factors that disrupt the brain's delicate equilibrium. This understanding has led to a shift in focus: from searching for one root cause to identifying how these elements interact to create a cascade of dysfunction.

At the heart of this synthesis is the concept of **systems failure**. The brain relies on tightly interconnected processes to maintain cognitive health, including synaptic communication, protein clearance, energy metabolism, and immune regulation. In Alzheimer's, these systems begin to fail, often subtly at first, with one dysfunction exacerbating another. For instance, amyloid plaques may trigger inflammation, which in turn disrupts mitochondrial function, leading to further neuronal damage and the spread of tau tangles. This interconnectedness makes Alzheimer's a self-perpetuating cycle that is difficult to halt once it begins.

The timing of these disruptions is also critical. Alzheimer's pathology can start decades before symptoms appear, highlighting the importance of early detection and intervention. Amyloid accumulation, for example, may act as an initial trigger, but its impact depends on other factors such as genetic risk, lifestyle, and systemic health. This explains why some individuals with significant amyloid buildup never develop cognitive decline, while others with minimal amyloid experience rapid progression.

One of the most transformative realizations has been the role of systemic health in Alzheimer's. Factors such as cardiovascular health, metabolic function, and chronic inflammation outside the brain significantly influence the risk and progression of the disease. This broader perspective shifts the focus from treating Alzheimer's as an isolated brain disease to addressing it as a systemic condition that reflects overall health.

Emerging research also highlights the importance of resilience—why some individuals are able to withstand significant brain pathology without noticeable cognitive decline. This concept, often referred to as **cognitive reserve**, underscores the protective role of lifestyle factors such as education, social engagement, and physical activity. It suggests that bolstering the brain's capacity to adapt and compensate is as important as addressing the pathology itself.

Synthesizing decades of evidence has revealed a more nuanced view of Alzheimer's: a disease driven by the interaction of multiple pathways rather than a single cause. This paradigm shift has profound implications for treatment and prevention. It emphasizes the need for a multifaceted approach that targets not just amyloid or tau but also inflammation, energy metabolism, vascular health, and lifestyle factors.

The pursuit of Alzheimer's root cause has evolved into a broader understanding of how the brain's systems break down over time. By integrating these insights, we are moving closer to a comprehensive model of the disease—one that acknowledges its complexity while providing actionable strategies for intervention.

As we continue to unravel this intricate web, one truth becomes clear: the future of Alzheimer's lies not in searching for one silver bullet but in addressing the many interconnected threads that contribute to its development. This synthesis of decades of evidence represents not just a scientific achievement but also a roadmap for hope, guiding us toward solutions that can preserve memory, identity, and the essence of what makes us human.

The Central Role of Chronic Inflammation

Chronic inflammation has emerged as a central player in the development and progression of Alzheimer's disease, bridging many of the pathological processes that define the condition. While inflammation is a natural and essential part of the body's immune response, its persistence over time can wreak havoc on the brain, setting the stage for neuronal dysfunction, cognitive decline, and the cascading effects of Alzheimer's pathology.

The Brain's Immune System

In the healthy brain, microglia, the resident immune cells, serve as sentinels that protect neurons by clearing away debris, damaged cells, and misfolded proteins such as amyloid-beta. Astrocytes, another type of glial cell, play a supportive role, maintaining the chemical environment and modulating immune activity. Together, these cells form the foundation of the brain's immune defense, ensuring a balanced response to potential threats.

In Alzheimer's disease, however, this balance is disrupted. Amyloid plaques, tau tangles, and other stressors trigger microglia and astrocytes to enter a prolonged state of activation. Initially, this activation is protective, aimed at containing the damage and clearing harmful proteins. But when the triggers persist, the immune response becomes chronic, resulting in the release of pro-inflammatory molecules such as cytokines and chemokines. These molecules, while intended to help, inadvertently cause collateral damage to healthy neurons and synapses.

Inflammation as a Driver of Alzheimer's

Chronic inflammation does more than amplify damage—it actively contributes to the progression of Alzheimer's. It impairs the brain's ability to clear amyloid-beta, leading to the accumulation of plaques. It also destabilizes tau proteins, promoting the formation of neurofibrillary tangles. Moreover, inflammation disrupts the blood-brain barrier, allowing harmful substances from the bloodstream to enter the brain and exacerbate the inflammatory response.

One of the most insidious effects of chronic inflammation is its impact on neuronal plasticity and communication. Pro-inflammatory cytokines interfere with synaptic signaling, impairing memory formation and cognitive function. Over time, the persistent inflammatory state accelerates neuronal loss, shrinking key regions of the brain, such as the hippocampus, which are critical for memory and learning.

Systemic Inflammation and Its Role

Chronic inflammation in Alzheimer's is not confined to the brain. Systemic inflammation—originating from conditions such as obesity, diabetes, cardiovascular disease, and autoimmune disorders—can cross the blood-brain barrier and fuel neuroinflammation. For instance, elevated levels of C-reactive protein (CRP), a marker of systemic inflammation, are associated with an increased risk of Alzheimer's.

Lifestyle factors also contribute to systemic inflammation. Diets high in processed foods and refined sugars promote inflammatory pathways, while physical inactivity, chronic stress, and poor sleep exacerbate systemic and neuroinflammation. These factors create a feedback loop where systemic inflammation intensifies neuroinflammation, accelerating Alzheimer's pathology.

Genetic Insights into Inflammation

Genetic studies have further highlighted the importance of inflammation in Alzheimer's. Variants in genes such as TREM2, which regulates microglial function, have been linked to an increased risk of Alzheimer's. These findings suggest that the brain's immune response is not only a consequence of the disease but a central driver of its progression.

Targeting Chronic Inflammation

Recognizing the central role of chronic inflammation has opened new avenues for treatment and prevention. Researchers are exploring drugs that can modulate the brain's immune response, shifting microglia and astrocytes from their harmful, overactive states to their protective roles. Anti-inflammatory compounds, such as nonsteroidal anti-inflammatory drugs (NSAIDs), have shown mixed results in clinical trials, but more targeted therapies, including monoclonal antibodies and small molecules, are showing promise in reducing neuroinflammation.

Beyond pharmaceuticals, lifestyle interventions offer significant potential for managing inflammation. Diets rich in anti-inflammatory compounds, such as the Mediterranean and MIND diets, can reduce systemic inflammation and promote brain health. Regular physical activity has been shown to modulate inflammatory markers, enhance neuroplasticity, and improve overall cognitive function. Practices like mindfulness meditation and stress reduction can also help lower levels of systemic inflammation, providing a holistic approach to managing Alzheimer's risk.

The Bigger Picture

Chronic inflammation is not just a byproduct of Alzheimer's—it is a central mechanism that ties together many of the disease's hallmark features. By understanding how inflammation fuels the pathology of Alzheimer's, we can target this process to interrupt the cycle of damage and progression.

As research continues to refine our understanding of inflammation's role, it becomes increasingly clear that addressing this factor is essential for effective treatment and prevention. Whether through targeted drugs, lifestyle changes, or systemic health improvements, reducing chronic inflammation offers a path toward preserving cognitive health and combating the devastating impact of Alzheimer's disease.

Ultimately, the central role of chronic inflammation underscores the interconnected nature of Alzheimer's and its systemic influences. By addressing this root cause, we take a crucial step toward unraveling the complexities of the disease and bringing hope to millions affected by its reach.

Part II: The Cure for Alzheimer's Disease

Chapter 6: The Holistic Approach to Healing

Why One-Size-Fits-All Treatments Fail

The search for a single, universal cure for Alzheimer's disease has dominated research for decades. From drugs targeting amyloid plaques to therapies aimed at tau tangles, the hope was that identifying the primary driver of the disease would lead to a straightforward solution. Yet, despite immense effort and investment, these approaches have largely fallen short of delivering the transformative outcomes patients and families so desperately need.

The failure of one-size-fits-all treatments lies in the very nature of Alzheimer's disease. Rather than being a singular condition with a uniform cause, Alzheimer's is a complex, multifaceted syndrome influenced by a wide range of biological, environmental, and lifestyle factors. Its variability among individuals underscores the need for a more nuanced and personalized approach to treatment.

The Complexity of Alzheimer's

Alzheimer's does not manifest the same way in every individual. Some patients may exhibit significant amyloid plaque buildup without experiencing cognitive decline, while others with minimal plaques may suffer from severe symptoms. Similarly, tau tangles, inflammation, vascular issues, and mitochondrial dysfunction contribute to the disease in different proportions for each person. This heterogeneity challenges the effectiveness of therapies that target only one aspect of the disease.

Genetic predisposition adds another layer of complexity. Variants such as APOE4 increase susceptibility, but even within this group, outcomes vary based on lifestyle, environmental exposures, and other genetic factors. For those without known genetic risk factors, the influence of systemic health, diet, exercise, and other external factors becomes even more pronounced.

The Problem with Singular Targets

Many of the most well-known Alzheimer's treatments have focused narrowly on amyloid-beta, operating under the assumption that reducing plaques would halt or reverse the disease. While these treatments have been successful in reducing amyloid levels, they have not consistently improved cognitive function or quality of life. This disconnect between the reduction of pathology and clinical outcomes highlights the limitations of a one-dimensional strategy.

Similarly, targeting tau tangles or inflammation in isolation has yielded mixed results. These approaches often fail to account for the interconnected nature of Alzheimer's pathology, where addressing one problem may leave others unaddressed—or even worsen them. For example, suppressing inflammation indiscriminately could impair the brain's natural repair mechanisms, while removing tau tangles might not address the underlying triggers that caused them to form in the first place.

The Importance of Individualized Treatment

Alzheimer's is best understood as a network problem—a disruption of multiple interconnected systems within the brain and body. Addressing one aspect of the disease without considering its broader context is akin to fixing one piece of a broken machine while ignoring the rest. Effective treatment requires a holistic approach that recognizes the unique combination of factors contributing to each patient's condition.

For example, a patient with Alzheimer's driven primarily by vascular dysfunction may benefit most from therapies that improve blood flow and cardiovascular health, while another patient with significant metabolic issues might respond better to dietary interventions or treatments targeting insulin resistance. Similarly, addressing systemic inflammation may be crucial for some individuals, whereas others might need therapies focused on mitochondrial function or oxidative stress.

Lessons from Other Chronic Conditions

The failure of one-size-fits-all treatments is not unique to Alzheimer's. Chronic diseases such as cancer, diabetes, and cardiovascular disease have shown that effective management often requires tailored strategies that address the patient's specific needs and circumstances. In oncology, for example, precision medicine has revolutionized treatment by matching therapies to the genetic and molecular profiles of individual tumors. A similar shift is needed in Alzheimer's care, where treatments are designed to target the unique constellation of factors driving each case.

The Path Forward

A holistic, individualized approach to Alzheimer's acknowledges that no single therapy will work for everyone. Instead, it combines multiple strategies, including:

- **Pharmacological treatments:** Targeting specific pathological mechanisms such as amyloid, tau, or inflammation.

- **Lifestyle modifications:** Promoting brain health through diet, exercise, stress management, and social engagement.

- **Systemic health interventions:** Addressing cardiovascular health, insulin resistance, and other metabolic factors.

- **Cognitive therapies:** Enhancing neuroplasticity through mental stimulation and memory exercises.

Advancements in biomarker testing, imaging, and genetic profiling are making it increasingly possible to tailor these interventions to the needs of individual patients. These tools allow clinicians to identify the primary drivers of Alzheimer's in each case and develop a personalized treatment plan.

A New Paradigm for Alzheimer's Care

The era of one-size-fits-all treatments is coming to an end, replaced by a more holistic and adaptive approach that reflects the complexity of Alzheimer's disease. This shift is not just about improving outcomes—it is about recognizing the individuality of each patient and addressing the unique factors that contribute to their condition.

By embracing this paradigm, we can move closer to a future where Alzheimer's is no longer a monolithic, untreatable disease but a condition that can be managed and even prevented through personalized, comprehensive care. This is the promise of the holistic approach to healing: a path that prioritizes the needs of the individual while leveraging the full spectrum of scientific and medical knowledge to combat one of humanity's greatest challenges.

Tailoring Solutions to Individual Needs

No two cases of Alzheimer's disease are exactly alike. While the disease is defined by common pathological features such as amyloid plaques and tau tangles, the underlying causes, progression, and manifestations vary widely from person to person. This variability makes it clear that a one-size-fits-all approach cannot adequately address the complexity of Alzheimer's. Instead, tailoring solutions to individual needs is essential for effective treatment and prevention.

Understanding Individual Variability

The variability in Alzheimer's arises from a multitude of factors, including genetics, lifestyle, comorbidities, and environmental exposures. For instance, a person with a genetic predisposition, such as carrying the APOE4 allele, may experience Alzheimer's differently than someone whose disease is primarily influenced by vascular or metabolic health. Similarly, a patient with significant inflammation may require a different therapeutic focus than one whose primary issue is mitochondrial dysfunction or oxidative stress.

This diversity is further reflected in the timing and progression of the disease. Some individuals exhibit mild cognitive impairment for years before advancing to dementia, while others experience rapid decline. These differences underscore the importance of identifying the unique combination of factors driving the disease in each individual.

Personalized Assessment

Tailoring solutions begins with a comprehensive assessment of each patient's condition. This includes:

1. **Genetic Testing:** Identifying risk genes such as APOE4 and other relevant mutations to understand genetic predisposition.

2. **Biomarker Analysis:** Measuring levels of amyloid-beta, tau, and other markers through cerebrospinal fluid or blood tests to pinpoint pathological changes.

3. **Neuroimaging:** Utilizing MRI or PET scans to evaluate brain atrophy, amyloid deposition, and other structural or functional changes.

4. **Lifestyle and Health History:** Examining factors such as diet, exercise habits, sleep quality, stress levels, and medical history to identify modifiable risk factors.

5. **Cognitive Testing:** Assessing memory, attention, and other cognitive functions to determine the current impact of the disease.

These tools provide a detailed picture of the patient's condition, allowing clinicians to identify the most relevant targets for intervention.

Personalized Treatment Plans

Once an individualized assessment is complete, a tailored treatment plan can be developed. This plan may include a combination of the following:

1. **Targeted Medications:** Depending on the patient's specific

pathology, drugs may be prescribed to address amyloid-beta, tau, inflammation, or other contributing factors. Emerging therapies, such as monoclonal antibodies or anti-inflammatory agents, may play a role in certain cases.

2. **Lifestyle Modifications:** Personalized recommendations for diet, exercise, and sleep are critical for optimizing brain health. For instance, a patient with insulin resistance may benefit from a low-glycemic or ketogenic diet, while one with vascular issues may focus on cardiovascular fitness.

3. **Cognitive Training:** Memory exercises, puzzles, and other cognitive therapies can be tailored to the patient's needs to enhance neuroplasticity and cognitive reserve.

4. **Mental and Emotional Support:** Addressing stress, anxiety, and depression through mindfulness, meditation, or therapy can help mitigate the effects of chronic stress on the brain.

5. **Social Engagement:** Encouraging meaningful social interactions can bolster cognitive resilience and improve overall quality of life.

6. **Comorbidities Management:** Treating coexisting conditions, such as hypertension, diabetes, or sleep apnea, is essential for reducing systemic inflammation and improving brain function.

Dynamic and Iterative Care

Personalized treatment for Alzheimer's is not a one-time process but a dynamic and iterative approach. As the disease progresses or as new information about the patient's condition emerges, the treatment plan must be adjusted. Regular monitoring of biomarkers, cognitive function, and overall health allows clinicians to refine interventions and address new challenges as they arise.

The Role of Technology

Advances in technology are making personalized care more accessible and precise. Wearable devices and apps can track activity levels, sleep quality, and vital signs, providing real-time feedback for patients and clinicians. AI-powered algorithms are being developed to analyze genetic, biomarker, and lifestyle data, offering tailored recommendations based on large datasets. These tools empower patients to take an active role in their care while enabling providers to deliver more targeted interventions.

Empowering Patients and Families

Tailoring solutions also involves empowering patients and their families to understand the disease and take control of the factors they can influence. Education about lifestyle modifications, stress management, and the importance of social and cognitive engagement can help patients and caregivers play an active role in treatment. Support networks and resources further enhance the capacity of families to manage the complexities of personalized care.

A Future of Personalized Alzheimer's Care

The move toward individualized treatment is a paradigm shift in Alzheimer's care. It recognizes that the disease is not a single entity but a collection of interrelated processes that manifest differently in each person. By tailoring solutions to individual needs, we not only improve outcomes but also honor the unique experiences of each patient.

This holistic and personalized approach offers a path forward—one where treatment is as diverse as the people it serves, and where hope is no longer limited by the confines of a single approach. It is through this commitment to individual care that we will unlock the full potential of healing and move closer to conquering Alzheimer's disease.

Chapter 7: Breakthrough Therapies

Targeting Amyloid and Tau Pathways

Amyloid plaques and tau tangles have long been central to our understanding of Alzheimer's disease. As the hallmarks of the condition, these pathological features have guided decades of research and therapeutic development. While early efforts to target amyloid and tau pathways faced numerous challenges, recent breakthroughs have brought new hope that these strategies can significantly slow or even halt the progression of Alzheimer's.

Targeting Amyloid Pathways

The amyloid-beta protein, a fragment of the amyloid precursor protein (APP), plays a critical role in the formation of plaques in Alzheimer's. These plaques disrupt neural communication and trigger inflammation, contributing to cognitive decline. Therapies aimed at amyloid have focused on reducing its production, enhancing its clearance, or preventing its aggregation.

1. **Reducing Amyloid Production**
   Drugs that inhibit beta-secretase and gamma-secretase enzymes, which are involved in the production of amyloid-beta, have been a focal point of research. Beta-secretase inhibitors, for example, aim to reduce the formation of amyloid-beta at its source. While early trials faced safety and efficacy issues, refinements in these therapies are showing promise in addressing the upstream production of amyloid-beta.

2. **Enhancing Amyloid Clearance**
   Monoclonal antibodies designed to tag amyloid-beta for removal by the immune system have gained significant traction. Drugs like aducanumab, lecanemab, and others in

development work by binding to amyloid plaques and facilitating their clearance by microglia, the brain's immune cells. While these therapies have demonstrated plaque reduction in clinical trials, their impact on cognitive outcomes has varied, emphasizing the need for early intervention and combination approaches.

3. **Preventing Amyloid Aggregation**
Small molecules that prevent amyloid-beta from clumping into plaques are another promising avenue. These therapies aim to stabilize amyloid-beta in its soluble form, reducing its toxicity and preventing the formation of insoluble deposits that disrupt brain function.

Targeting Tau Pathways

While amyloid-beta is often seen as an initiator of Alzheimer's pathology, tau tangles are closely linked to the disease's progression and cognitive decline. Tau, a protein that stabilizes the brain's transport structures, becomes hyperphosphorylated in Alzheimer's, leading to its aggregation into neurofibrillary tangles. Therapies targeting tau aim to prevent its abnormal modifications, reduce its accumulation, or block its spread.

1. **Preventing Tau Phosphorylation**
Inhibitors of kinases such as GSK-3β, which phosphorylate tau, are being developed to prevent the formation of abnormal tau. These drugs aim to restore normal tau function and reduce the formation of tangles.

2. **Clearing Abnormal Tau**
Similar to amyloid-targeting therapies, monoclonal antibodies are being used to target tau. These antibodies bind to pathological tau and promote its clearance from the brain. Early trials suggest that such therapies may slow cognitive decline by reducing the burden of tau tangles.

3. **Blocking Tau Propagation**
Recent discoveries have revealed that misfolded tau can spread between neurons, propagating the disease throughout the brain. Small molecules and antibodies that

block this spread are a promising new approach, aiming to contain the damage and prevent further neuronal loss.

Combining Amyloid and Tau Therapies

One of the most exciting developments in Alzheimer's research is the growing recognition that amyloid and tau are interconnected and that effective treatment may require addressing both pathways. Amyloid accumulation often precedes tau pathology, suggesting that early amyloid-targeting therapies could prevent or delay tau-related damage. Conversely, targeting tau in later stages may mitigate the symptoms caused by neuronal dysfunction.

Combination therapies that address both amyloid and tau simultaneously or sequentially are being explored. These strategies acknowledge the complexity of Alzheimer's and aim to tackle multiple facets of the disease for a more comprehensive approach.

Challenges and Opportunities

While therapies targeting amyloid and tau pathways represent a significant leap forward, they are not without challenges. Many treatments are most effective in the early stages of the disease, highlighting the importance of early diagnosis and intervention. Furthermore, individual variability in response to these therapies underscores the need for personalized approaches that consider genetic, environmental, and systemic factors.

Another challenge is balancing efficacy and safety. Some amyloid-targeting therapies have been associated with side effects such as brain swelling or microbleeds, requiring careful monitoring during treatment. Researchers are continually refining these therapies to minimize risks while maximizing benefits.

A New Era of Alzheimer's Treatment

Breakthroughs in targeting amyloid and tau pathways mark the beginning of a new era in Alzheimer's treatment. These therapies offer hope that we can slow or halt the disease's progression, particularly when combined with early detection and lifestyle interventions. They also pave the way for further innovations, including the integration of anti-inflammatory, metabolic, and vascular strategies to address the broader context of Alzheimer's pathology.

As research continues to advance, the promise of amyloid and tau therapies is becoming a reality. These breakthroughs bring us closer to transforming Alzheimer's from an incurable condition into one that can be effectively managed, giving patients and their families hope for a brighter future.

The Role of Anti-Inflammatory Drugs

The recognition of chronic inflammation as a central driver of Alzheimer's disease has sparked significant interest in the potential of anti-inflammatory drugs to mitigate its effects. Neuroinflammation, while initially a protective response, becomes destructive when sustained, contributing to neuronal damage, amyloid accumulation, and tau pathology. As a result, targeting inflammation offers a promising avenue for slowing or even halting the progression of Alzheimer's.

The Mechanisms of Neuroinflammation

In Alzheimer's, the brain's immune cells—primarily microglia and astrocytes—become hyperactivated in response to amyloid plaques, tau tangles, and other stressors. This activation leads to the release of pro-inflammatory molecules such as cytokines and chemokines. While these molecules are intended to combat damage, prolonged activation creates a toxic environment that exacerbates neuronal dysfunction and impairs the brain's ability to clear amyloid-beta and other harmful substances.

Anti-inflammatory drugs aim to disrupt this harmful cycle by modulating the immune response, reducing the production of inflammatory molecules, or restoring the brain's immune balance.

Nonsteroidal Anti-Inflammatory Drugs (NSAIDs)

NSAIDs, such as ibuprofen and aspirin, have been widely studied for their potential role in Alzheimer's prevention and treatment.

These drugs inhibit cyclooxygenase (COX) enzymes, reducing the production of prostaglandins, which are mediators of inflammation. Observational studies have suggested that long-term NSAID use may reduce the risk of Alzheimer's, particularly in individuals with genetic risk factors such as the APOE4 allele.

However, clinical trials of NSAIDs for treating Alzheimer's have yielded mixed results. While they may be effective in reducing inflammation in the early stages of the disease, their benefits appear limited once Alzheimer's pathology has progressed. Additionally, prolonged NSAID use carries risks, including gastrointestinal and cardiovascular side effects, making their widespread application in Alzheimer's treatment challenging.

Selective Anti-Inflammatory Drugs

The limitations of traditional NSAIDs have led to the development of more selective anti-inflammatory drugs that target specific pathways involved in neuroinflammation. For example:

- **PDE4 Inhibitors:** These drugs reduce the production of pro-inflammatory cytokines by targeting phosphodiesterase 4 (PDE4), an enzyme involved in inflammatory signaling. Early studies suggest they may reduce inflammation without the side effects associated with NSAIDs.

- **NLRP3 Inflammasome Inhibitors:** The NLRP3 inflammasome is a protein complex that amplifies the inflammatory response in the brain. Drugs targeting this pathway aim to curb excessive immune activation while preserving protective functions.

- **Microglial Modulators:** Therapies that shift microglia from their pro-inflammatory state to a neuroprotective state are showing promise in preclinical studies. These drugs may help clear amyloid-beta and reduce neuronal damage.

Immunomodulatory Approaches

Beyond traditional anti-inflammatory drugs, immunomodulatory therapies are being explored to fine-tune the brain's immune response. For instance:

- **Cytokine Inhibitors:** Drugs that block specific cytokines, such as interleukin-1β (IL-1β) or tumor necrosis factor-alpha (TNF-α), are being tested for their ability to reduce harmful inflammation without suppressing the entire immune system.
- **Monoclonal Antibodies:** Antibodies targeting inflammatory molecules or receptors, such as TREM2, are designed to regulate microglial activity and restore balance to the brain's immune environment.

The Timing of Intervention

One of the key lessons from anti-inflammatory research is the importance of timing. Chronic inflammation often begins years before symptoms of Alzheimer's emerge, suggesting that early intervention may be critical. Anti-inflammatory therapies are likely to be most effective in the preclinical or early stages of the disease, when inflammation has not yet caused widespread neuronal damage.

Lifestyle and Anti-Inflammatory Strategies

While pharmacological approaches hold promise, lifestyle interventions that reduce systemic and neuroinflammation can complement drug therapies. Diets rich in anti-inflammatory foods, such as the Mediterranean or MIND diets, provide nutrients that support brain health. Regular physical activity reduces systemic inflammation and promotes neurogenesis, while stress reduction techniques, such as mindfulness and meditation, can lower inflammatory markers. These strategies may enhance the effectiveness of anti-inflammatory drugs and provide a foundation for prevention.

Challenges and Future Directions

Developing effective anti-inflammatory drugs for Alzheimer's presents several challenges. The brain's immune system is highly complex, and suppressing inflammation indiscriminately can impair its protective functions. The blood-brain barrier also limits the delivery of many drugs, requiring innovative approaches to ensure that treatments reach their target.

Despite these challenges, ongoing research is identifying new pathways and targets for anti-inflammatory therapies. Advances in biomarkers and neuroimaging are enabling more precise monitoring of inflammation, allowing researchers to tailor treatments to individual patients and stages of the disease.

A Promising Path Forward

The role of chronic inflammation in Alzheimer's is undeniable, and anti-inflammatory drugs represent a critical component of the therapeutic arsenal. By modulating the brain's immune response, these therapies have the potential to slow the progression of Alzheimer's and improve quality of life for millions of patients.

When combined with other approaches that address amyloid, tau, and systemic factors, anti-inflammatory drugs could pave the way for a comprehensive treatment strategy that targets the disease from multiple angles. As research continues to advance, the promise of these therapies brings us closer to a future where the destructive effects of neuroinflammation can be controlled, offering hope for those affected by Alzheimer's and their families.

Cutting-Edge Gene Therapy

Gene therapy is at the forefront of medical innovation, offering transformative possibilities for treating complex diseases like Alzheimer's. By directly modifying the genetic material within cells, gene therapy aims to address the root causes of the disease rather than merely alleviating its symptoms. Recent breakthroughs in gene-editing technologies and delivery systems have opened new avenues for targeting the genetic and molecular drivers of Alzheimer's, providing hope for more precise and effective treatments.

The Promise of Gene Therapy in Alzheimer's

Alzheimer's has a strong genetic component, with certain genes significantly influencing the risk and progression of the disease. While rare mutations in genes like **APP, PSEN1,** and **PSEN2** cause early-onset familial Alzheimer's, more common variants, such as **APOE4,** increase the risk of late-onset Alzheimer's. Gene therapy offers the potential to modify or silence these harmful genes, enhance the expression of protective ones, or repair faulty genetic instructions.

In addition to targeting genetic risk factors, gene therapy can also address other aspects of Alzheimer's pathology, such as amyloid-beta production, tau phosphorylation, and neuroinflammation. By delivering therapeutic genes directly to affected brain regions, this approach allows for localized and sustained intervention.

Strategies in Gene Therapy

1. **Gene Silencing and Editing**
    - **CRISPR-Cas9 Technology:** CRISPR-Cas9 is a powerful tool for editing DNA. In Alzheimer's, it can be used to silence genes that produce harmful proteins, such as amyloid-beta. For example, researchers are exploring ways to disrupt the activity of beta-secretase (BACE1), an enzyme involved in amyloid-beta production, without affecting other critical cellular functions.
    - **RNA Interference (RNAi):** RNAi uses small RNA molecules to silence specific genes by preventing their translation into proteins. This approach is being investigated to reduce the production of tau or amyloid-beta, targeting these proteins at their source.

2. **Gene Replacement**
    - Gene replacement therapy introduces functional copies of genes to compensate for defective or mutated ones. For familial Alzheimer's caused by mutations in APP or PSEN genes, replacing the faulty gene with a healthy version could prevent or

delay the onset of the disease.

3. **Enhancing Protective Genes**
   - Certain genes, such as **APOE2,** are associated with a reduced risk of Alzheimer's. Gene therapy could be used to introduce APOE2 into individuals carrying the high-risk APOE4 variant, potentially mitigating their genetic risk. This strategy aims to tilt the balance toward neuroprotection rather than neurodegeneration.

4. **Neurotrophic Factor Delivery**
   - Gene therapy can be used to deliver neurotrophic factors—proteins that support neuron survival and repair. For example, genes encoding brain-derived neurotrophic factor (BDNF) or nerve growth factor (NGF) can be introduced into affected brain regions to promote neuronal health and resilience, countering the effects of Alzheimer's pathology.

Advances in Gene Delivery Systems

One of the critical challenges in gene therapy is ensuring that therapeutic genes reach their target without causing off-target effects. Advances in delivery systems are making this goal increasingly achievable:

- **Viral Vectors:** Modified viruses, such as adeno-associated viruses (AAVs), are commonly used to deliver therapeutic genes. These vectors can be engineered to target specific brain cells and regions, minimizing the risk of unintended effects.

- **Non-Viral Methods:** Emerging technologies, such as nanoparticles and liposomes, offer non-viral alternatives for delivering genetic material. These methods are less likely to provoke immune responses and can be tailored for precise targeting.

- **Intrathecal and Intravenous Delivery:** Innovative delivery routes, such as injecting gene therapies directly into the cerebrospinal fluid (intrathecal delivery) or bloodstream, are being explored to enhance accessibility and effectiveness.

Challenges and Ethical Considerations

Despite its promise, gene therapy for Alzheimer's faces several challenges:

- **Delivery to the Brain:** The blood-brain barrier limits the entry of therapeutic agents, requiring advanced strategies to ensure effective delivery.
- **Long-Term Effects:** The durability and safety of gene edits over time remain uncertain, necessitating rigorous long-term studies.
- **Ethical Concerns:** Gene therapy raises ethical questions, particularly regarding the potential for germline editing (modifications passed to future generations) and the equitable distribution of high-cost treatments.

Current Progress and Future Directions

Several gene therapy approaches for Alzheimer's are in preclinical or early clinical trial stages. These include therapies targeting tau, amyloid-beta, and neuroinflammation, as well as those aimed at enhancing neuroprotection. Early results are encouraging, demonstrating the potential to slow or reverse disease progression.

The future of gene therapy in Alzheimer's lies in its integration with other treatment modalities. For instance, combining gene therapy with anti-inflammatory drugs, amyloid-targeting monoclonal antibodies, or lifestyle interventions could offer a comprehensive approach to managing the disease.

A Paradigm Shift in Treatment

Gene therapy represents a paradigm shift in Alzheimer's treatment, focusing on precision and personalization. By addressing the root causes of the disease at a molecular level, it offers the potential for long-lasting and transformative effects. While the road to widespread implementation is still under construction, the progress made thus far suggests that gene therapy could play a pivotal role in the fight against Alzheimer's.

As research continues, the promise of gene therapy brings hope not only for halting the progression of Alzheimer's but also for fundamentally altering its trajectory. It is a testament to the power of innovation and a glimpse into a future where this devastating disease may one day be consigned to history.

Chapter 8: The Nutritional Connection

Diet's Role in Brain Health

The old adage "you are what you eat" has profound implications when it comes to brain health, particularly in the context of Alzheimer's disease. Emerging research highlights the critical role of diet in maintaining cognitive function, reducing the risk of neurodegenerative diseases, and even influencing the progression of Alzheimer's. While genetics and other factors play significant roles, nutrition is one of the most modifiable elements of brain health, offering a powerful tool for prevention and treatment.

The Brain's Nutritional Needs

The human brain, despite accounting for only about 2% of body weight, consumes approximately 20% of the body's energy. Its high metabolic demands require a steady supply of nutrients to maintain cellular function, support neurotransmitter synthesis, and protect against oxidative stress and inflammation. Deficiencies in key nutrients can impair these processes, leaving the brain vulnerable to damage and accelerating the progression of conditions like Alzheimer's.

Key nutrients for brain health include:

- **Omega-3 Fatty Acids:** Found in fatty fish, flaxseeds, and walnuts, omega-3s, particularly DHA, are essential for maintaining the structural integrity of neuronal membranes and supporting synaptic function.

- **Antioxidants:** Vitamins C and E, along with polyphenols in foods like berries, green tea, and dark chocolate, combat oxidative stress, a major contributor to Alzheimer's pathology.

- **B Vitamins:** Vitamins B6, B12, and folate play critical roles in reducing homocysteine levels, an amino acid associated with cognitive decline when elevated.
- **Vitamin D:** Linked to neuroprotection and reduced inflammation, vitamin D deficiency is a risk factor for cognitive impairment.

Diet and Cognitive Decline

The connection between diet and Alzheimer's has been underscored by numerous studies, which reveal that certain dietary patterns can either increase or decrease the risk of cognitive decline.

1. **The Standard Western Diet**

   Diets high in refined sugars, saturated fats, and processed foods have been linked to inflammation, insulin resistance, and oxidative stress, all of which contribute to Alzheimer's pathology. The Western diet's nutrient-poor and calorie-dense nature promotes systemic and neuroinflammation, accelerating cognitive decline.

2. **Protective Diets**

   In contrast, diets emphasizing whole, nutrient-dense foods have been shown to protect brain health. Two of the most studied diets in this context are:

   - **The Mediterranean Diet:** Rich in fruits, vegetables, whole grains, lean proteins (particularly fish), and healthy fats like olive oil, this diet has consistently been associated with reduced risk of Alzheimer's and slower cognitive decline.
   - **The MIND Diet (Mediterranean-DASH Intervention for Neurodegenerative Delay):** A hybrid of the Mediterranean and DASH (Dietary Approaches to Stop Hypertension) diets, the MIND diet specifically targets brain health by emphasizing foods such as leafy greens, berries, nuts, and fish

while limiting red meat, butter, and sugary foods.

Mechanisms Linking Diet to Alzheimer's

The protective effects of a healthy diet stem from its ability to address key mechanisms underlying Alzheimer's pathology:

- **Reducing Inflammation:** Anti-inflammatory foods, such as those rich in omega-3 fatty acids and polyphenols, help counteract chronic inflammation in the brain, which contributes to amyloid and tau pathology.

- **Enhancing Glymphatic Clearance:** Nutrient-rich diets promote the glymphatic system, which removes toxins like amyloid-beta during sleep.

- **Improving Insulin Sensitivity:** Diets low in refined sugars and high in fiber help regulate blood sugar levels and reduce insulin resistance, a condition linked to Alzheimer's.

- **Protecting Against Oxidative Stress:** Antioxidant-rich foods neutralize free radicals, preventing oxidative damage to neurons.

Practical Dietary Recommendations

Incorporating brain-healthy foods into daily life doesn't require a complete dietary overhaul. Small, sustainable changes can have a significant impact:

- **Prioritize Healthy Fats:** Replace saturated fats with unsaturated options like olive oil, avocados, and nuts.

- **Increase Fish Consumption:** Aim for at least two servings of fatty fish, such as salmon or sardines, per week.

- **Embrace Colorful Produce:** Eat a variety of fruits and vegetables, focusing on dark leafy greens and vibrant berries.

- **Choose Whole Grains:** Replace refined carbohydrates with whole grains like quinoa, oats, and brown rice.

- **Limit Processed Foods:** Reduce intake of processed

snacks, sugary drinks, and fast foods.
- **Stay Hydrated:** Adequate hydration is crucial for maintaining cognitive function.

The Future of Nutrition in Alzheimer's Care

As research into the nutritional connection to Alzheimer's evolves, personalized nutrition plans based on genetic, metabolic, and lifestyle factors may become a key component of treatment. Advances in nutrigenomics—the study of how genes interact with diet—are helping identify individual dietary needs, enabling tailored interventions to maximize brain health.

Beyond Food

While diet is a cornerstone of brain health, it is most effective when combined with other lifestyle factors such as regular exercise, quality sleep, and stress management. These complementary strategies amplify the benefits of a brain-healthy diet, creating a holistic approach to Alzheimer's prevention and care.

A Path to Empowerment

Diet's role in brain health offers a message of empowerment: through conscious food choices, individuals can take proactive steps to protect their cognitive function and reduce their risk of Alzheimer's. By focusing on nourishing the brain with the right nutrients, we can support its resilience and unlock a future where Alzheimer's is not an inevitability but a preventable and manageable condition.

Nutraceuticals That Support Cognitive Function

Nutraceuticals—dietary supplements or food-derived compounds that offer health benefits beyond basic nutrition—have gained attention as potential tools in the fight against Alzheimer's disease. These compounds, often derived from plants, vitamins, minerals, and other natural sources, target the biological pathways underlying cognitive decline. By addressing oxidative stress, inflammation, mitochondrial dysfunction, and more, nutraceuticals hold promise as adjuncts to traditional treatments and lifestyle interventions.

The Science Behind Nutraceuticals

The brain's high energy demands and vulnerability to oxidative stress make it particularly reliant on compounds that protect against damage and support cellular function. Nutraceuticals, with their antioxidant, anti-inflammatory, and neuroprotective properties, can bolster the brain's defenses and enhance resilience against Alzheimer's pathology.

While no single nutraceutical can cure Alzheimer's, emerging research suggests that a combination of these compounds may support cognitive function and slow disease progression. Below are some of the most promising nutraceuticals for brain health:

Omega-3 Fatty Acids

- **Source:** Found in fish oil, flaxseed, and walnuts.
- **Mechanism:** Omega-3s, particularly DHA (docosahexaenoic acid), are critical for maintaining neuronal membrane integrity and reducing neuroinflammation. They also promote synaptic plasticity, essential for learning and memory.
- **Evidence:** Studies show that higher omega-3 intake is associated with reduced amyloid deposition and slower cognitive decline.

Curcumin

- **Source:** Derived from turmeric, curcumin is a potent antioxidant and anti-inflammatory compound.
- **Mechanism:** Curcumin reduces oxidative stress and inhibits the aggregation of amyloid-beta and tau proteins. It

also enhances the clearance of amyloid plaques by stimulating microglial activity.
- **Evidence:** Clinical trials suggest that curcumin may improve memory and attention in older adults, though its bioavailability (absorption) remains a challenge. Formulations with enhanced bioavailability are under development.

Resveratrol

- **Source:** Found in red wine, grapes, and peanuts.
- **Mechanism:** Resveratrol activates sirtuins, proteins involved in cellular repair and longevity. It also enhances mitochondrial function, reduces neuroinflammation, and improves blood-brain barrier integrity.
- **Evidence:** Preliminary studies indicate that resveratrol supplementation may slow cognitive decline and reduce markers of neurodegeneration.

B Vitamins

- **Source:** Found in fortified cereals, leafy greens, meat, and eggs.
- **Mechanism:** Vitamins B6, B12, and folate help lower homocysteine levels, an amino acid associated with cognitive decline and brain atrophy.
- **Evidence:** Clinical trials have shown that B vitamin supplementation can slow brain shrinkage in regions critical for memory, particularly in individuals with high homocysteine levels.

Phosphatidylserine (PS)

- **Source:** A phospholipid found in soybeans and other foods.
- **Mechanism:** PS supports the structural integrity of neuronal membranes and facilitates synaptic communication. It also plays a role in reducing cortisol levels, which may help mitigate stress-related cognitive decline.
- **Evidence:** Studies suggest that PS supplementation improves memory and attention, particularly in early cognitive impairment.

Coenzyme Q10 (CoQ10)

- **Source:** Naturally occurring in the body and found in foods like fish, meat, and nuts.
- **Mechanism:** CoQ10 supports mitochondrial function and reduces oxidative damage by neutralizing free radicals.
- **Evidence:** Although research in Alzheimer's is limited, CoQ10 has shown promise in protecting neurons and supporting energy metabolism.

Ginkgo Biloba

- **Source:** Extracted from the leaves of the ginkgo tree.
- **Mechanism:** Ginkgo biloba enhances blood flow to the brain, reduces oxidative stress, and protects against neuronal damage.
- **Evidence:** Clinical studies show mixed results, but some suggest modest improvements in memory and executive function, particularly in individuals with mild cognitive impairment.

Polyphenols

- **Source:** Found in berries, green tea, dark chocolate, and coffee.

- **Mechanism:** Polyphenols are powerful antioxidants that combat oxidative stress and modulate inflammatory pathways. Specific compounds, such as EGCG (epigallocatechin gallate) in green tea, have neuroprotective effects.
- **Evidence:** Regular consumption of polyphenol-rich foods is associated with better cognitive performance and reduced risk of dementia.

Vitamin D

- **Source:** Sunlight exposure and fortified foods.
- **Mechanism:** Vitamin D supports calcium homeostasis, reduces inflammation, and promotes neuronal health.
- **Evidence:** Low vitamin D levels are associated with an increased risk of Alzheimer's, and supplementation may improve cognitive outcomes in deficient individuals.

Practical Considerations

Quality and Dosage: Nutraceuticals vary widely in quality and potency. Choosing high-quality, clinically tested supplements is essential for safety and efficacy.

Synergistic Effects: Combining multiple nutraceuticals with complementary mechanisms may enhance their effectiveness. For example, omega-3s and antioxidants like curcumin and resveratrol may work together to reduce inflammation and oxidative stress.

Timing: Nutraceuticals may be most effective in the early stages of Alzheimer's or as preventive measures, emphasizing the importance of early intervention.

The Future of Nutraceuticals

The field of nutraceutical research is rapidly evolving, with advancements in delivery systems and formulations enhancing their bioavailability and efficacy. Personalized nutrition, guided by genetic and biomarker analysis, may further optimize the use of nutraceuticals by tailoring interventions to individual needs.

As part of a holistic approach to Alzheimer's prevention and treatment, nutraceuticals complement dietary, lifestyle, and pharmacological strategies. While they are not a standalone cure, their ability to support cognitive function and promote brain health makes them a valuable component in the fight against Alzheimer's.

By integrating these natural compounds into a broader plan for brain health, we can empower individuals to take proactive steps toward preserving memory and cognitive resilience, offering hope in the battle against this devastating disease.

The Ketogenic Diet and Beyond

Among the various dietary approaches explored for Alzheimer's prevention and management, the ketogenic diet has garnered significant attention. Originally developed to treat epilepsy, this high-fat, low-carbohydrate diet is now being studied for its potential neuroprotective effects in Alzheimer's disease. By altering the brain's primary energy source, the ketogenic diet may address key mechanisms of the disease, including energy deficits, inflammation, and oxidative stress.

The Science Behind the Ketogenic Diet

The ketogenic diet works by shifting the body's metabolism from glucose to ketones as its primary energy source. Ketones, produced in the liver during the breakdown of fats, are a highly efficient fuel for the brain. In Alzheimer's, the brain's ability to metabolize glucose is impaired—a condition known as cerebral glucose hypometabolism—which contributes to cognitive decline. Ketones bypass this dysfunction, providing an alternative energy source that supports neuronal health and function.

Mechanisms of the Ketogenic Diet in Alzheimer's

Improved Energy Metabolism

Ketones restore energy production in neurons, compensating for glucose metabolism deficits. This improved energy supply helps maintain synaptic activity and cognitive function.

Reduction in Inflammation

The ketogenic diet reduces systemic and neuroinflammation by modulating inflammatory pathways and decreasing the production of pro-inflammatory cytokines.

Protection Against Oxidative Stress

Ketones enhance mitochondrial function and reduce the generation of reactive oxygen species (ROS), which cause oxidative damage in the brain.

Enhanced Clearance of Amyloid-Beta

Animal studies suggest that a ketogenic diet may promote the clearance of amyloid-beta by enhancing glymphatic system activity and reducing its accumulation in the brain.

Improved Insulin Sensitivity

Insulin resistance is a common feature in Alzheimer's, often referred to as "type 3 diabetes." The ketogenic diet improves insulin sensitivity and reduces hyperinsulinemia, mitigating its effects on brain health.

Evidence Supporting the Ketogenic Diet

Research on the ketogenic diet and Alzheimer's is still in its early stages, but the findings are promising:

Animal Studies: Preclinical research shows that ketogenic diets improve cognitive function, reduce amyloid-beta accumulation, and protect against neuronal loss in Alzheimer's models.

Human Trials: Preliminary trials suggest that ketogenic diets or ketone supplements (such as medium-chain triglycerides, MCTs) improve memory, attention, and executive function in individuals with mild cognitive impairment (MCI) or early Alzheimer's.

Challenges and Considerations

Adherence: The strict dietary restrictions of the ketogenic diet—limiting carbohydrates to less than 10% of daily calories—can be challenging to maintain for many individuals.

Safety: Long-term adherence to a ketogenic diet may have side effects, including nutrient deficiencies, gastrointestinal issues, and increased cardiovascular risk in some individuals. Monitoring by healthcare professionals is essential.

Personalization: Not all individuals respond equally to ketogenic diets. Genetic factors, metabolic health, and disease stage may influence its effectiveness.

Expanding Beyond Ketosis

While the ketogenic diet holds promise, it is not the only dietary approach with potential benefits for Alzheimer's. Other strategies can complement or serve as alternatives:

Intermittent Fasting: Periodic fasting or time-restricted eating mimics some effects of the ketogenic diet by promoting ketone production, improving insulin sensitivity, and reducing inflammation.

Mediterranean Diet with MCTs: Combining the well-established benefits of the Mediterranean diet with MCT oil supplementation offers a more flexible approach to ketone production.

Low-Glycemic Diets: Diets that limit refined carbohydrates and sugars stabilize blood glucose levels, reduce insulin resistance, and mitigate inflammation.

Plant-Based Diets: Diets rich in plant-based foods provide antioxidants, fiber, and anti-inflammatory compounds, supporting overall brain health.

Future Directions

Research into the ketogenic diet and related dietary approaches is expanding, with an emphasis on optimizing protocols for Alzheimer's prevention and treatment. Combining ketogenic strategies with other interventions, such as exercise, nutraceuticals, and pharmacological therapies, may amplify their effects.

Additionally, advancements in personalized nutrition are enabling the development of tailored dietary plans based on genetic and metabolic profiles, ensuring that individuals receive the most effective intervention for their unique needs.

A Balanced Perspective

The ketogenic diet and its derivatives represent exciting tools in the nutritional arsenal against Alzheimer's, but they are not a universal solution. They are most effective when integrated into a broader, holistic approach that includes other lifestyle modifications, medical treatments, and support systems.

By exploring the ketogenic diet and beyond, we open new doors to understanding how nutrition shapes brain health and how dietary strategies can empower individuals to take control of their cognitive well-being. This evolving field holds immense potential for reshaping the future of Alzheimer's care, offering hope for prevention and improved quality of life.

Chapter 9: Restoring the Brain's Ecosystem

Gut-Brain Axis: The Forgotten Frontier

In recent years, the relationship between the gut and the brain has emerged as one of the most fascinating and transformative areas of neuroscience. Known as the **gut-brain axis**, this bidirectional communication network links the central nervous system with the gastrointestinal system, revealing the profound influence that gut health has on brain function. In the context of Alzheimer's disease, disruptions in this axis are increasingly recognized as significant contributors to cognitive decline, inflammation, and neurodegeneration.

The Gut as a "Second Brain"

The gut is often referred to as the body's "second brain" due to its extensive network of neurons, neurotransmitter production, and ability to communicate with the brain via the vagus nerve and systemic pathways. It also houses the gut microbiome, a diverse community of trillions of microorganisms that play critical roles in digestion, immune regulation, and metabolic processes.

How the Gut Affects the Brain

Microbiome Composition and Cognitive Health

The balance of beneficial and harmful bacteria in the gut microbiome profoundly influences brain health. Dysbiosis, or an imbalance in the microbiome, has been linked to systemic inflammation, increased permeability of the intestinal barrier ("leaky gut"), and heightened risk of Alzheimer's.

Beneficial bacteria produce short-chain fatty acids (SCFAs) like butyrate, which have anti-inflammatory and neuroprotective properties. Conversely, harmful bacteria can release toxins and pro-inflammatory molecules that disrupt neuronal function.

Immune System Modulation

The gut is home to 70% of the body's immune cells, making it a central hub for immune regulation. Dysbiosis can trigger chronic low-grade inflammation, which can cross the blood-brain barrier and contribute to neuroinflammation, a key driver of Alzheimer's pathology.

Metabolic and Neurotransmitter Production

The gut microbiome produces metabolites and neurotransmitters such as serotonin, dopamine, and gamma-aminobutyric acid (GABA), which influence mood, cognition, and overall brain function. Disruptions in these pathways can impair communication between the gut and brain.

Amyloid Production and Clearance

Some gut bacteria are capable of producing amyloid-like proteins, which may mimic or exacerbate the formation of amyloid-beta in the brain. Dysbiosis can also interfere with the brain's ability to clear amyloid plaques, compounding the effects of Alzheimer's.

Evidence Linking the Gut-Brain Axis to Alzheimer's

Emerging research underscores the importance of the gut-brain axis in Alzheimer's:

Gut Dysbiosis in Alzheimer's Patients: Studies have shown that individuals with Alzheimer's have altered microbiome compositions, with reduced levels of beneficial bacteria like **Bifidobacterium** and **Lactobacillus** and increased levels of harmful bacteria associated with inflammation.

Leaky Gut and Neuroinflammation: Intestinal permeability, or "leaky gut," allows toxins and inflammatory molecules to enter the bloodstream, crossing the blood-brain barrier and triggering neuroinflammation.

Animal Models: Preclinical studies have demonstrated that restoring a healthy microbiome in animal models of Alzheimer's reduces amyloid-beta accumulation, improves cognitive function, and decreases inflammation.

Restoring Balance: Strategies for the Gut-Brain Axis

Dietary Interventions

A diet rich in fiber, prebiotics, and probiotics supports a healthy microbiome. Foods like fermented vegetables, yogurt, and high-fiber plants promote the growth of beneficial bacteria and the production of SCFAs.

Reducing processed foods, sugar, and artificial additives minimizes the proliferation of harmful bacteria and inflammation-promoting compounds.

Probiotic and Prebiotic Supplements

Probiotics are live beneficial bacteria that can restore microbial balance, while prebiotics are non-digestible fibers that feed these bacteria. Supplements targeting specific strains associated with brain health, such as **Lactobacillus plantarum** and **Bifidobacterium longum**, show promise in reducing inflammation and improving cognition.

Fecal Microbiota Transplantation (FMT)

Though still experimental, FMT involves transferring gut microbiota from a healthy donor to a patient. Early studies suggest it may improve cognitive outcomes by restoring microbiome diversity.

Polyphenols and Natural Compounds

Compounds found in green tea, berries, and dark chocolate support gut health by promoting beneficial bacteria and reducing oxidative stress. These polyphenols also have neuroprotective properties.

Stress Reduction and the Vagus Nerve

Chronic stress negatively impacts the gut microbiome and weakens the gut-brain connection. Practices like mindfulness, yoga, and deep breathing stimulate the vagus nerve, enhancing communication between the gut and brain while reducing inflammation.

The Future of Gut-Brain Research in Alzheimer's

The gut-brain axis is reshaping how we view Alzheimer's disease, shifting the focus from isolated brain pathology to the broader ecosystem that supports cognitive health. Ongoing research aims to develop microbiome-based diagnostics and targeted therapies, such as custom probiotic formulations or dietary protocols tailored to individual microbiome profiles.

By addressing gut health, we not only mitigate risk factors for Alzheimer's but also open new pathways for prevention and treatment. This "forgotten frontier" holds immense potential to complement existing therapies and unlock deeper insights into the interconnected systems that sustain brain health.

Restoring the gut-brain axis is not just about improving digestion—it is about creating a foundation for cognitive resilience and overall well-being. As we continue to explore this frontier, we move closer to a future where Alzheimer's is better understood, more effectively managed, and ultimately preventable.

Detoxifying the Brain: The Role of Sleep and Glymphatic Drainage

Sleep is often referred to as the brain's housekeeping period, and for good reason. During this crucial state of rest, the brain engages in essential processes that help maintain its health and function. Among the most vital of these is the activity of the **glymphatic system**, a specialized waste clearance mechanism that removes toxins, including amyloid-beta and tau, the hallmark proteins associated with Alzheimer's disease. Disruptions in sleep and glymphatic function can lead to an accumulation of these harmful substances, contributing to cognitive decline and neurodegeneration.

The Glymphatic System: The Brain's Cleaning Crew

The glymphatic system, discovered in 2012, is a network of channels that facilitates the removal of metabolic waste from the brain. It operates most efficiently during sleep, using cerebrospinal fluid (CSF) to flush toxins and debris from the brain's interstitial spaces. The system relies on the coordinated activity of glial cells, particularly astrocytes, which help regulate the flow of CSF and interstitial fluid.

During sleep, the brain undergoes structural changes that enhance glymphatic activity. Neuronal activity decreases, allowing astrocytes to expand the spaces between cells, increasing fluid flow and waste clearance. This process is particularly effective at removing amyloid-beta, whose buildup forms the plaques characteristic of Alzheimer's.

The Link Between Sleep and Alzheimer's

Numerous studies have established a strong connection between sleep disturbances and Alzheimer's:

Amyloid and Sleep Disruption: Poor sleep quality or insufficient sleep increases amyloid-beta levels, while elevated amyloid levels can, in turn, disrupt sleep patterns, creating a vicious cycle.

Tau Accumulation: Sleep deprivation accelerates the accumulation of tau protein, which forms neurofibrillary tangles that impair neuronal communication.

Sleep Architecture: Disruptions in deep sleep stages, particularly slow-wave sleep (SWS), are associated with reduced glymphatic activity and impaired toxin clearance.

Sleep Disorders and Cognitive Decline

Sleep disorders, such as insomnia, sleep apnea, and restless leg syndrome, are common in individuals with Alzheimer's and may contribute to disease progression:

Obstructive Sleep Apnea (OSA): OSA reduces oxygen levels in the brain and disrupts sleep cycles, impairing glymphatic function and promoting inflammation. Treating OSA with continuous positive airway pressure (CPAP) therapy has been shown to improve cognitive outcomes.

Chronic Insomnia: Persistent difficulty falling or staying asleep can exacerbate amyloid and tau accumulation, increasing the risk of cognitive decline.

Strategies to Enhance Sleep and Glymphatic Function

Restoring healthy sleep patterns and optimizing glymphatic drainage are key components of a holistic approach to Alzheimer's prevention and management.

Establish a Sleep-Friendly Environment

Maintain a consistent sleep schedule, aiming for 7–9 hours of quality sleep per night.

Create a dark, quiet, and cool bedroom environment to promote deep sleep.

Prioritize Slow-Wave Sleep

Engage in activities that promote slow-wave sleep, such as moderate aerobic exercise and mindfulness practices. Deep sleep is essential for glymphatic activity and memory consolidation.

Treat Sleep Disorders

Address underlying sleep disorders, such as sleep apnea, with appropriate therapies like CPAP. Consulting a sleep specialist can help identify and manage sleep-related issues.

Support the Glymphatic System

Sleep Position: Sleeping on one's side (lateral position) has been shown to enhance glymphatic efficiency compared to sleeping on the back or stomach.

Hydration: Adequate hydration supports CSF production, which is critical for glymphatic function.

Avoiding Alcohol and Sedatives: Excessive alcohol and sedative use can disrupt sleep architecture and impair glymphatic clearance.

Diet and Timing

Avoid heavy meals and caffeine close to bedtime to minimize disruptions to sleep quality.

Consider a diet rich in antioxidants and anti-inflammatory foods to support overall brain health.

Enhance Circadian Rhythms

Exposure to natural light during the day and avoiding blue light from screens before bed helps regulate circadian rhythms, promoting better sleep.

The Broader Implications of Sleep and Glymphatic Health

The role of sleep and glymphatic drainage in Alzheimer's extends beyond toxin clearance. These processes are also critical for synaptic plasticity, memory consolidation, and overall brain health. Chronic sleep disturbances can exacerbate systemic inflammation, insulin resistance, and oxidative stress, all of which are contributors to Alzheimer's pathology.

Recognizing sleep as a cornerstone of brain health underscores the importance of integrating sleep hygiene into preventive and therapeutic strategies for Alzheimer's. As research continues to uncover the intricacies of the glymphatic system, new interventions—such as drugs that enhance glymphatic flow or devices that stimulate specific sleep stages—may become powerful tools in combating Alzheimer's.

A Path to Restoration

Improving sleep quality and glymphatic function offers a practical and accessible way to support brain health and reduce Alzheimer's risk. By prioritizing these aspects of the brain's ecosystem, we can help detoxify the mind, preserve cognitive function, and create a foundation for resilience against neurodegeneration. Sleep is not just a passive state; it is an active, vital process for protecting the brain and fostering long-term health.

Supporting Neurogenesis

Neurogenesis, the process of generating new neurons, was once thought to cease after early development. However, groundbreaking research has revealed that the brain retains the ability to produce new neurons well into adulthood, particularly in the hippocampus, a region critical for memory and learning. This discovery has significant implications for Alzheimer's disease, as enhancing neurogenesis may help counteract neuronal loss and support cognitive resilience.

In Alzheimer's, the hippocampus is one of the first areas to be affected, leading to memory impairment and difficulty forming new memories. Supporting neurogenesis offers a pathway to restore and maintain the brain's capacity for adaptation and repair, potentially slowing or reversing the progression of the disease.

The Role of Neurogenesis in Brain Health

Neurogenesis contributes to brain health in several ways:

Memory Formation: Newly formed neurons integrate into existing neural circuits, enhancing the brain's capacity to store and retrieve information.

Cognitive Flexibility: Neurogenesis supports the brain's ability to adapt to new information and environments, a critical function for problem-solving and learning.

Repair and Recovery: New neurons can replace those lost to injury, disease, or aging, helping maintain neural network integrity.

In Alzheimer's, the decline in neurogenesis contributes to cognitive deficits and the brain's reduced ability to recover from damage. Enhancing neurogenesis may provide a means to mitigate these effects.

Strategies to Support Neurogenesis

Physical Exercise

Regular aerobic exercise, such as walking, running, or swimming, is one of the most effective ways to boost neurogenesis. Exercise increases levels of brain-derived neurotrophic factor (BDNF), a protein that promotes the growth and survival of new neurons.

Studies show that physically active individuals have larger hippocampal volumes and better cognitive function, even in later life.

Nutritional Support

Omega-3 Fatty Acids: Found in fatty fish and flaxseeds, omega-3s, particularly DHA, are essential for neuronal membrane formation and neurogenesis.

Polyphenols: Compounds in foods like berries, green tea, and dark chocolate support neurogenesis by reducing inflammation and oxidative stress.

Curcumin: This compound, derived from turmeric, enhances BDNF levels and promotes the proliferation of neural stem cells.

Cognitive Stimulation

Engaging in mentally stimulating activities, such as learning a new skill, solving puzzles, or playing musical instruments, encourages the integration of new neurons into existing networks.

Cognitive training exercises tailored to memory, reasoning, and problem-solving can enhance hippocampal function.

Stress Reduction

Chronic stress and elevated cortisol levels suppress neurogenesis, particularly in the hippocampus. Stress reduction techniques, such as mindfulness, meditation, and yoga, can protect and support neuronal growth.

Sleep Optimization

Quality sleep is essential for neurogenesis. During slow-wave sleep, the brain consolidates memories and clears toxins, creating an optimal environment for new neurons to thrive. Maintaining a regular sleep schedule and addressing sleep disorders can enhance this process.

Intermittent Fasting and Caloric Restriction

Intermittent fasting and moderate caloric restriction have been shown to stimulate neurogenesis by increasing BDNF levels and enhancing metabolic efficiency. These dietary strategies may also reduce inflammation and oxidative stress, supporting overall brain health.

Pharmacological Interventions

Emerging therapies aim to directly enhance neurogenesis by targeting molecular pathways such as BDNF signaling or the proliferation of neural stem cells. While still experimental, these treatments hold promise for augmenting the brain's capacity for repair and adaptation.

The Challenges of Enhancing Neurogenesis

While the potential of neurogenesis in Alzheimer's is exciting, it is not without challenges:

Integration into Neural Circuits: New neurons must integrate seamlessly into existing networks to provide meaningful cognitive benefits. This process requires precise coordination of growth, survival, and synaptic connectivity.

Balancing Other Pathologies: Enhancing neurogenesis alone may not address other aspects of Alzheimer's pathology, such as amyloid accumulation, tau tangles, and inflammation. A comprehensive approach is necessary.

The Future of Neurogenesis Research

Ongoing research seeks to better understand the mechanisms of neurogenesis and how they can be harnessed for therapeutic benefit. Advances in stem cell technology, gene editing, and neurotrophic factor delivery are paving the way for innovative interventions. For example, transplanting neural stem cells or stimulating endogenous stem cells in the brain could provide new avenues for restoring lost function in Alzheimer's patients.

A Holistic Approach to Neurogenesis

Supporting neurogenesis is not a standalone solution but a vital part of a broader strategy to restore the brain's ecosystem. By combining lifestyle modifications, dietary interventions, and emerging therapies, we can create an environment that fosters neuronal growth and resilience.

Neurogenesis represents hope in the face of neuronal loss—a testament to the brain's remarkable capacity for regeneration. By nurturing this process, we take an essential step toward preserving memory, cognition, and the essence of what makes us human in the fight against Alzheimer's disease.

Chapter 10: Lifestyle Medicine

Exercise as Medicine for the Brain

Exercise is one of the most powerful and accessible interventions for promoting brain health and combating Alzheimer's disease. Far from being just a tool for physical fitness, regular physical activity profoundly impacts the brain, influencing its structure, function, and resilience against neurodegeneration. Research consistently shows that exercise is not just preventive—it can actively enhance cognitive function and slow the progression of Alzheimer's in those already affected.

The Neuroscience of Exercise

Exercise exerts its benefits on the brain through multiple mechanisms, including:

Increased Neurogenesis

Exercise stimulates the production of new neurons, particularly in the hippocampus, a region critical for memory and learning. This neurogenic effect is mediated by the release of brain-derived neurotrophic factor (BDNF), a protein that supports neuronal growth, survival, and plasticity.

Enhanced Synaptic Plasticity

Physical activity strengthens existing synaptic connections and promotes the formation of new ones, improving the brain's ability to adapt and store information.

Improved Cerebral Blood Flow

Exercise increases blood flow to the brain, delivering oxygen and nutrients while facilitating the removal of waste products such as amyloid-beta.

Reduction in Neuroinflammation

Regular physical activity reduces the production of pro-inflammatory cytokines, mitigating the chronic inflammation that contributes to Alzheimer's pathology.

Mitochondrial Health

Exercise enhances mitochondrial function and energy production in brain cells, reducing oxidative stress and supporting cellular resilience.

Stress Regulation

By lowering cortisol levels, exercise helps counteract the negative effects of chronic stress on the hippocampus and other brain regions.

Evidence Supporting Exercise in Alzheimer's

Numerous studies underscore the impact of exercise on brain health:

Preventive Effects: Longitudinal studies show that individuals who engage in regular physical activity are less likely to develop Alzheimer's. Aerobic exercise, in particular, has been associated with a reduced risk of cognitive decline.

Cognitive Benefits: In individuals with mild cognitive impairment (MCI), exercise has been shown to improve memory, attention, and executive function, delaying progression to Alzheimer's.

Structural Changes: Imaging studies reveal that exercise increases hippocampal volume and preserves gray matter, counteracting the atrophy commonly seen in Alzheimer's.

Types of Exercise and Their Benefits

Not all exercise is created equal, and different types of physical activity offer unique benefits for brain health:

Aerobic Exercise

Activities such as walking, running, swimming, and cycling are particularly effective at improving cardiovascular fitness and cerebral blood flow. They also boost BDNF levels, supporting neurogenesis and synaptic plasticity.

Resistance Training

Weightlifting and resistance exercises improve strength and mobility while enhancing cognitive function. These exercises increase levels of insulin-like growth factor 1 (IGF-1), which supports brain plasticity and repair.

Mind-Body Exercises

Practices such as yoga, tai chi, and Pilates combine physical movement with mindfulness, reducing stress and improving overall brain function. These exercises are particularly beneficial for individuals who may have difficulty engaging in high-intensity workouts.

Balance and Coordination Activities

Exercises like dancing and martial arts challenge the brain to integrate multiple sensory inputs, enhancing cognitive flexibility and neural connectivity.

How Much Exercise Is Enough?

The optimal "dose" of exercise for brain health depends on individual factors, but general guidelines suggest:

Frequency: At least 150 minutes of moderate-intensity aerobic exercise per week, spread across multiple sessions.

Intensity: Activities that elevate the heart rate and induce mild sweating are most effective. For individuals with limited mobility, even light activities such as walking or chair exercises provide benefits.

Duration: Sessions lasting 30–60 minutes are ideal for promoting sustained physiological effects on the brain.

Overcoming Barriers to Exercise

For many individuals, particularly those with Alzheimer's or mobility challenges, starting and maintaining an exercise routine can be daunting. Strategies to overcome barriers include:

Starting Small: Begin with low-intensity activities, such as short walks, and gradually increase duration and intensity.

Incorporating Social Interaction: Group classes or exercise partners provide motivation and social engagement, both of which enhance adherence and brain health.

Personalized Programs: Tailor exercises to the individual's abilities and preferences to ensure safety and enjoyment.

Professional Guidance: Physical therapists and fitness trainers can design customized programs for those with specific needs or limitations.

Exercise as Part of a Comprehensive Strategy

While exercise alone cannot cure Alzheimer's, it is a cornerstone of a broader lifestyle medicine approach that includes nutrition, sleep optimization, cognitive stimulation, and stress management. Together, these interventions create a synergistic effect, amplifying the benefits of each individual component.

The Hope in Motion

Exercise is a powerful tool for promoting cognitive resilience, protecting against neurodegeneration, and improving quality of life. It is a prescription for both prevention and healing, offering hope to individuals at risk of or living with Alzheimer's. By incorporating regular physical activity into daily life, we can empower individuals to take control of their brain health and move toward a brighter, more active future.

Stress Reduction and Mindfulness

Chronic stress is a silent contributor to many diseases, and Alzheimer's is no exception. Persistent stress can impair memory, accelerate cognitive decline, and exacerbate the progression of neurodegenerative diseases. The link between stress and Alzheimer's lies in its impact on brain regions like the hippocampus, systemic inflammation, and overall brain resilience. Stress reduction techniques and mindfulness practices offer a powerful means to counteract these effects, fostering a healthier brain environment and enhancing cognitive function.

The Impact of Stress on the Brain

Hippocampal Atrophy

Chronic stress leads to elevated levels of cortisol, a stress hormone that, in excess, damages neurons in the hippocampus. Since the hippocampus is essential for memory and learning, this damage accelerates cognitive decline and increases vulnerability to Alzheimer's.

Increased Inflammation

Stress triggers the release of pro-inflammatory cytokines, which can cross the blood-brain barrier and contribute to neuroinflammation, a key driver of Alzheimer's pathology.

Impaired Neurogenesis

Stress suppresses the production of new neurons in the hippocampus, limiting the brain's ability to adapt and recover from damage.

Disrupted Sleep

Chronic stress often interferes with sleep, reducing the brain's ability to clear toxins like amyloid-beta and undermining cognitive health.

The Role of Stress Reduction

Reducing stress not only mitigates these harmful effects but also promotes resilience and cognitive function. Stress reduction techniques are especially valuable for individuals at risk of or living with Alzheimer's, as they address both the physiological and emotional aspects of the disease.

Mindfulness and Its Benefits

Mindfulness is the practice of focusing attention on the present moment with a sense of openness and acceptance. It has been shown to reduce stress, enhance emotional regulation, and improve overall well-being. For brain health, mindfulness offers specific benefits:

Lowered Cortisol Levels: Regular mindfulness practice reduces cortisol and other stress hormones, protecting the hippocampus from stress-related damage.

Enhanced Neuroplasticity: Mindfulness promotes the growth of new neural connections, supporting cognitive flexibility and learning.

Improved Sleep: Mindfulness practices, such as meditation, have been shown to improve sleep quality, enhancing the brain's detoxification processes.

Reduced Inflammation: Mindfulness has anti-inflammatory effects, reducing the chronic low-grade inflammation that contributes to Alzheimer's pathology.

Stress Reduction Techniques

Meditation

Practices like mindfulness meditation, transcendental meditation, and guided imagery can calm the mind, reduce stress hormones, and enhance focus and memory.

Even short daily sessions of 10–20 minutes can yield significant benefits.

Deep Breathing Exercises

Techniques such as diaphragmatic breathing or the 4-7-8 method activate the parasympathetic nervous system, promoting relaxation and reducing stress.

Yoga and Tai Chi

These mind-body practices combine physical movement with

mindfulness, reducing stress while improving flexibility, balance, and strength. They also support better sleep and mood regulation.

Progressive Muscle Relaxation (PMR)

PMR involves tensing and relaxing muscle groups in sequence, promoting physical and mental relaxation. It can be particularly effective for managing stress and improving sleep.

Journaling

Expressive writing about thoughts and feelings can help process stress and foster emotional clarity. Journaling gratitude or positive experiences also enhances well-being.

Social Connection

Building and maintaining strong social bonds can reduce feelings of isolation and stress. Supportive relationships are associated with improved cognitive resilience and overall health.

Creating a Mindful Routine

Integrating stress reduction and mindfulness practices into daily life doesn't require dramatic changes. Small, consistent habits can have profound effects:

Start the day with 5–10 minutes of meditation or deep breathing.

Incorporate mindfulness into everyday activities, such as eating, walking, or even doing chores.

Set aside time for a yoga or tai chi class a few times a week.

Dedicate a few minutes before bed to journaling or guided relaxation.

The Long-Term Benefits

The cumulative effects of stress reduction and mindfulness extend beyond immediate relaxation. Over time, these practices enhance emotional resilience, improve memory and attention, and protect the brain from age-related decline. For individuals with Alzheimer's, mindfulness can also help manage anxiety, depression, and agitation, improving quality of life for both patients and caregivers.

A Holistic Approach to Brain Health

Stress reduction and mindfulness are integral components of a holistic approach to Alzheimer's care. When combined with exercise, nutrition, and cognitive engagement, these practices create a supportive environment for brain health and cognitive resilience.

By learning to manage stress and cultivate mindfulness, individuals take an active role in preserving their cognitive function and emotional well-being. These practices not only protect the brain but also foster a sense of calm and empowerment, offering hope in the face of life's challenges.

Social Engagement and Cognitive Resilience

Human beings are inherently social creatures, and the quality of our relationships and interactions profoundly affects brain health. In the context of Alzheimer's disease, social engagement plays a critical role in building cognitive resilience—the brain's ability to adapt and compensate for damage. Research consistently shows that maintaining meaningful social connections can protect against cognitive decline, slow the progression of Alzheimer's, and enhance overall well-being.

The Link Between Social Engagement and Brain Health

Cognitive Stimulation

Social interactions challenge the brain by requiring attention, memory, language, and problem-solving skills. These activities strengthen neural connections and promote cognitive flexibility.

Neuroplasticity

Meaningful social interactions encourage the formation of new neural pathways, supporting the brain's ability to adapt and recover from damage.

Reduced Stress and Inflammation

Strong social bonds reduce levels of cortisol, the stress hormone that can harm the hippocampus. Social engagement also mitigates systemic inflammation, a key contributor to Alzheimer's pathology.

Emotional Support

Positive social connections foster a sense of belonging and purpose, reducing the risk of depression and anxiety, which are known to exacerbate cognitive decline.

Evidence Supporting Social Engagement

Numerous studies highlight the protective effects of social engagement:

Reduced Risk of Dementia: Individuals with robust social networks are significantly less likely to develop Alzheimer's compared to those who are socially isolated.

Slower Cognitive Decline: Active social engagement has been associated with slower rates of memory loss and better executive function in older adults.

Increased Longevity: Socially connected individuals tend to live longer, with better overall health and quality of life.

Strategies for Enhancing Social Engagement

For those at risk of or living with Alzheimer's, fostering social connections can be an empowering step toward building cognitive resilience. Here are some practical strategies:

Join Community Activities

Participating in group activities such as book clubs, exercise classes, or art workshops encourages interaction and cognitive engagement.

Volunteer

Volunteering provides a sense of purpose and facilitates meaningful connections with others. It also promotes regular social interaction, a key factor in maintaining cognitive health.

Maintain Family and Friend Relationships

Regularly connecting with loved ones through visits, phone calls, or video chats helps reinforce emotional bonds and keeps the mind active.

Engage in Intergenerational Activities

Spending time with younger generations, such as grandchildren, fosters mental stimulation and emotional fulfillment. Activities like storytelling, board games, or shared hobbies create opportunities for cognitive engagement.

Participate in Cognitive or Creative Group Activities

Group settings for activities like music therapy, dance, or memory games combine social interaction with cognitive stimulation, enhancing their benefits.

Technology for Connection

For those with limited mobility or geographic constraints, technology can facilitate social engagement through video calls, social media, or online discussion forums.

Overcoming Barriers to Social Engagement

Challenges such as physical limitations, hearing loss, or social anxiety can hinder participation in social activities. Addressing these barriers is crucial:

Address Mobility Issues: Transportation services, community programs, or virtual events can provide accessible options.

Support Hearing or Vision Needs: Hearing aids, assistive devices, or well-lit environments can enhance communication and participation.

Foster Safe Spaces: Creating inclusive and welcoming environments encourages individuals to engage without fear of judgment or discomfort.

The Role of Caregivers and Communities

Caregivers and community members play a vital role in fostering social engagement for individuals with Alzheimer's:

Caregiver Involvement: Caregivers can facilitate participation in social activities, provide encouragement, and ensure that interactions are positive and meaningful.

Community Programs: Initiatives such as memory cafés, support groups, and dementia-friendly events provide opportunities for individuals to connect and engage in a supportive setting.

A Holistic Approach to Social Connection

Social engagement should be integrated into a broader lifestyle approach to Alzheimer's prevention and management, complementing other strategies such as physical activity, nutrition, and cognitive training. Together, these interventions create a synergistic effect, maximizing cognitive resilience and overall well-being.

Social Bonds as a Source of Strength

The power of social connection lies in its ability to nourish both the mind and the soul. For individuals facing Alzheimer's, meaningful relationships provide not only a source of cognitive stimulation but also a foundation of emotional support and hope. By prioritizing social engagement, we can foster a sense of belonging, strengthen cognitive resilience, and create a brighter future for those affected by this challenging disease.

Part III: Preventing Alzheimer's

Chapter 11: Risk Reduction Strategies

Early Detection and Biomarkers

Alzheimer's disease often begins its destructive course decades before noticeable symptoms emerge. This long preclinical phase presents a critical window for intervention, during which early detection could significantly alter the trajectory of the disease. Biomarkers—biological indicators of disease processes—are at the forefront of this effort, enabling the identification of Alzheimer's risk and progression long before cognitive decline becomes apparent. By leveraging these tools, clinicians and researchers can target prevention strategies and tailor interventions to those who stand to benefit most.

The Importance of Early Detection

Preventative Interventions

Identifying individuals at risk for Alzheimer's during the preclinical stage allows for the implementation of lifestyle modifications, pharmacological therapies, and other interventions to delay or prevent disease onset.

Personalized Treatment

Biomarkers enable a more precise understanding of the underlying pathology, allowing treatments to be tailored to the specific needs of each patient.

Monitoring Progression

Early detection tools provide a baseline for tracking disease progression, helping clinicians evaluate the effectiveness of interventions and adjust strategies as needed.

Key Biomarkers for Alzheimer's Disease

Amyloid-Beta and Tau Proteins

Amyloid-Beta: The buildup of amyloid plaques is a hallmark of Alzheimer's. Abnormal levels of amyloid-beta can be detected in cerebrospinal fluid (CSF) and, more recently, through blood-based assays.

Tau: Hyperphosphorylated tau protein forms tangles within neurons, contributing to cognitive decline. Elevated tau levels in CSF or the presence of tau pathology via PET imaging indicate ongoing neurodegeneration.

Neurodegeneration Markers

Neurofilament Light Chain (NfL): NfL is a protein released when neurons are damaged. Its presence in blood or CSF serves as a marker of neurodegeneration and disease progression.

Brain Atrophy: MRI imaging reveals structural changes, such as hippocampal atrophy, that correlate with cognitive decline.

Inflammatory Markers

Chronic neuroinflammation plays a central role in Alzheimer's. Biomarkers like C-reactive protein (CRP) and cytokines (e.g., IL-6, TNF-alpha) provide insights into the inflammatory environment contributing to disease pathology.

Genetic Markers

APOE Genotyping: The APOE4 allele is the strongest genetic risk factor for late-onset Alzheimer's. Genetic testing can identify carriers who may benefit from targeted prevention strategies.

Rare Mutations: Mutations in APP, PSEN1, or PSEN2 genes indicate familial Alzheimer's, though these cases are rare.

Metabolic and Vascular Markers

Conditions like insulin resistance, elevated blood glucose, and vascular dysfunction increase Alzheimer's risk. Biomarkers such as HbA1c (glycated hemoglobin) and cholesterol levels provide a broader picture of systemic health and its impact on the brain.

Advances in Biomarker Technology

Recent breakthroughs in biomarker research are transforming Alzheimer's detection and monitoring:

Blood-Based Biomarkers

Historically, biomarker detection required invasive procedures like lumbar punctures or expensive imaging technologies. Blood-based biomarkers, such as plasma amyloid-beta and phosphorylated tau, are revolutionizing accessibility, offering cost-effective and minimally invasive options.

Neuroimaging

Advanced imaging techniques, including PET scans and functional MRI (fMRI), allow for the visualization of amyloid plaques, tau tangles, and changes in brain activity. These tools provide critical insights into the disease's progression.

Digital Biomarkers

Wearable devices and smartphone applications are emerging as tools for monitoring subtle changes in cognition, sleep, and physical activity, offering early warning signs of cognitive decline.

Artificial Intelligence (AI)

AI algorithms can analyze complex biomarker data, identifying patterns and predicting disease risk with remarkable accuracy. AI also aids in interpreting neuroimaging and other diagnostic tools.

Challenges in Early Detection

Despite these advances, several challenges remain:

Ethical Considerations: Early diagnosis may raise concerns about the psychological impact of knowing one's risk and the potential for discrimination in insurance or employment.

False Positives/Negatives: Biomarkers are not perfect predictors, and misinterpretation could lead to unnecessary anxiety or missed opportunities for intervention.

Access and Equity: High costs and limited availability of advanced diagnostic tools may restrict access for certain populations.

The Future of Early Detection

The integration of biomarkers into routine clinical practice has the potential to transform Alzheimer's care. As diagnostic tools become more accessible and accurate, they will enable:

Precision Medicine: Treatments tailored to the specific biomarkers driving an individual's disease.

Wider Preventative Screening: Routine biomarker testing in midlife could identify at-risk individuals long before symptoms arise.

Real-Time Monitoring: Advances in wearable technology and remote monitoring will allow for continuous assessment of brain health, enabling timely interventions.

Empowering Prevention Through Awareness

Early detection empowers individuals to take proactive steps to protect their brain health. With knowledge of their risk, they can adopt lifestyle modifications, participate in clinical trials, and engage in targeted therapies designed to delay or prevent the onset of Alzheimer's.

A New Era in Alzheimer's Prevention

Biomarkers are ushering in a new era of Alzheimer's prevention and treatment. By identifying the disease at its earliest stages, we can intervene before irreversible damage occurs, offering hope for millions of individuals and their families. Early detection is not just a diagnostic breakthrough—it is a beacon of possibility, guiding us toward a future where Alzheimer's is preventable and manageable.

Personalized Preventative Plans

No two individuals experience Alzheimer's disease in the same way, and the factors that contribute to its onset and progression vary widely. As such, a personalized approach to prevention is essential. By tailoring interventions to an individual's genetic, lifestyle, and environmental risk factors, personalized preventative plans provide a proactive framework for reducing the likelihood of cognitive decline and maintaining brain health.

The Need for Personalization

Diverse Risk Profiles

Genetic predisposition, such as carrying the **APOE4** allele, significantly increases Alzheimer's risk for some individuals, while others may be more affected by lifestyle factors like poor diet, sedentary behavior, or chronic stress. Personalized plans address these unique profiles.

Disease Heterogeneity

Alzheimer's encompasses a spectrum of underlying pathologies, including amyloid plaques, tau tangles, neuroinflammation, and vascular dysfunction. A one-size-fits-all approach cannot effectively address this complexity.

Modifiable Risk Factors

Up to 40% of Alzheimer's cases are thought to be influenced by modifiable risk factors, highlighting the potential for individualized interventions to make a meaningful difference.

Steps to Create a Personalized Plan

Comprehensive Assessment

Genetic Testing: Identifying genetic risks, such as **APOE4** or familial Alzheimer's mutations, provides a foundation for tailoring interventions.

Biomarker Analysis: Blood or cerebrospinal fluid tests can reveal amyloid-beta levels, tau, inflammation markers, and other indicators of brain health.

Lifestyle Evaluation: Assessing diet, physical activity, sleep quality, stress levels, and social engagement identifies areas for improvement.

Medical History: Chronic conditions such as diabetes, hypertension, and depression are significant contributors to Alzheimer's risk and must be factored into the plan.

Targeted Lifestyle Modifications

Diet: Tailor dietary recommendations to the individual's metabolic needs and preferences. For instance, individuals with insulin resistance may benefit from a low-glycemic or ketogenic diet, while others may thrive on the Mediterranean or MIND diet.

Exercise: Develop an exercise regimen based on fitness level, mobility, and interests, incorporating aerobic, resistance, and mind-body practices.

Sleep: Address sleep disorders or habits that impair rest, such as untreated sleep apnea or poor sleep hygiene.

Stress Management and Mental Health Support

Integrate mindfulness practices, meditation, or therapy to address chronic stress and mental health concerns, tailoring methods to the individual's comfort and responsiveness.

Cognitive Engagement

Provide personalized recommendations for intellectually stimulating activities, such as puzzles, reading, or learning a new skill, based on the individual's interests and cognitive strengths.

Social Engagement

Encourage participation in social activities that align with the individual's personality and preferences, such as volunteering, group classes, or family gatherings.

Addressing Comorbidities

Collaborate with healthcare providers to manage chronic conditions that exacerbate Alzheimer's risk, such as cardiovascular disease, diabetes, and depression.

Tools for Implementation

Digital Health Technologies

Apps and wearable devices can monitor activity, sleep, heart rate, and cognitive performance, providing real-time feedback and encouraging adherence.

Regular Check-Ins

Schedule periodic evaluations to monitor progress, adjust strategies, and address new challenges. Biomarker tests and cognitive assessments can track improvements or detect early signs of decline.

Support Systems

Engage family members, caregivers, and social networks to provide accountability, motivation, and emotional support.

Challenges and Considerations

Accessibility and Equity

Personalized plans must account for socioeconomic disparities, ensuring access to diagnostic tools, healthy foods, and exercise opportunities.

Motivation and Adherence

Behavioral change can be challenging. Providing education, incremental goals, and consistent encouragement increases the likelihood of sustained adherence.

Ethical Implications

Genetic and biomarker testing raises concerns about psychological impact, privacy, and potential misuse of data. Informed consent and counseling are essential components of ethical implementation.

The Benefits of Personalization

Proactive Prevention

Personalized plans empower individuals to take control of their brain health, targeting risk factors before symptoms appear.

Enhanced Effectiveness

Tailored strategies address the unique needs of each individual, maximizing the potential for meaningful outcomes.

Quality of Life

By focusing on holistic health, personalized plans improve not only cognitive resilience but also overall well-being.

A Model for Future Prevention

Personalized preventative plans represent the future of Alzheimer's care, integrating advances in genetic, biomarker, and lifestyle research to offer targeted, effective solutions. These plans shift the focus from reactive treatment to proactive prevention, enabling individuals to live longer, healthier lives with their cognitive abilities intact.

As the science of Alzheimer's prevention continues to evolve, personalized approaches will play a central role in reducing the burden of this devastating disease, offering hope and empowerment to millions around the world.

Chapter 12: Building a Brain-Healthy World

Policies for Public Health

The fight against Alzheimer's disease extends beyond individual prevention and treatment—it is a societal challenge requiring comprehensive public health strategies. As the global population ages and the prevalence of Alzheimer's increases, policies aimed at fostering a brain-healthy environment have never been more critical. Public health initiatives can reduce risk factors, promote early detection, and ensure equitable access to care, creating a world better equipped to combat Alzheimer's.

The Need for Public Health Policies

Global Burden of Alzheimer's

Alzheimer's is not only a personal tragedy but also a societal one, imposing immense economic, emotional, and healthcare burdens. By 2050, the number of people living with Alzheimer's is projected to triple, straining healthcare systems and caregivers worldwide.

Modifiable Risk Factors

Up to 40% of Alzheimer's cases are linked to modifiable risk factors, such as physical inactivity, poor diet, and social isolation. Public health policies targeting these factors offer a significant opportunity for prevention.

Health Disparities

Socioeconomic inequalities contribute to disparities in Alzheimer's risk and care. Policies must address these gaps to ensure that all individuals have access to prevention and treatment resources.

Key Policy Areas

Education and Awareness

Public Awareness Campaigns: Increase understanding of Alzheimer's risk factors, early symptoms, and the importance of prevention through nationwide campaigns.

Brain Health Education: Integrate brain health into school curriculums, emphasizing lifelong habits that reduce the risk of cognitive decline.

Caregiver Support Resources: Provide education for caregivers on managing Alzheimer's and maintaining their own mental and physical health.

Access to Preventative Care

Routine Screening Programs: Encourage early detection through regular cognitive assessments in primary care, especially for at-risk populations.

Subsidized Biomarker Testing: Make diagnostic tools, such as blood tests and imaging, affordable and accessible to all.

Lifestyle Intervention Programs: Develop community-based programs offering free or low-cost resources for exercise, nutrition, and stress management.

Healthy Food Policies

Incentives for Nutritious Foods: Subsidize fruits, vegetables, and whole grains to make brain-healthy diets more affordable.

Regulation of Processed Foods: Reduce the availability of processed foods high in sugar and unhealthy fats, which contribute to cognitive decline.

Public Nutrition Programs: Expand initiatives like school lunch programs to include brain-boosting foods, ensuring all children have access to a healthy diet.

Promoting Physical Activity

Infrastructure for Exercise: Build accessible walking paths, bike lanes, and parks to encourage physical activity.

Workplace Wellness Programs: Incentivize employers to provide exercise opportunities, such as gym memberships or on-site fitness classes.

Targeted Community Programs: Offer free exercise classes tailored to older adults and those with limited mobility.

Social Engagement and Cognitive Health

Community Centers and Programs: Fund spaces and activities that promote social connection, such as senior centers, memory cafés, and intergenerational events.

Combatting Loneliness: Support initiatives that address social isolation, particularly in older adults, through outreach programs and volunteer opportunities.

Research and Innovation

Increased Funding for Alzheimer's Research: Prioritize investment in understanding the disease's causes, developing treatments, and improving diagnostic tools.

Collaborative Efforts: Promote public-private partnerships to accelerate research and innovation.

Global Knowledge Sharing: Encourage international collaboration to share insights, strategies, and breakthroughs.

Policy Challenges

Economic Constraints

Implementing large-scale public health initiatives requires significant investment, which may be challenging for resource-limited regions. Policies should emphasize cost-effectiveness and prioritize high-impact interventions.

Behavioral Change

Encouraging individuals to adopt healthier lifestyles requires overcoming deeply ingrained habits and cultural norms. Education campaigns must be culturally sensitive and tailored to diverse populations.

Healthcare System Limitations

Many healthcare systems lack the infrastructure to deliver widespread preventive care and early detection services. Policies should focus on building capacity and integrating brain health into primary care.

A Global Call to Action

Alzheimer's is a global challenge requiring coordinated efforts across nations and sectors. Organizations like the World Health Organization (WHO) and Alzheimer's Disease International (ADI) play critical roles in driving global initiatives, such as the WHO's Global Action Plan on Dementia, which emphasizes prevention, diagnosis, and care.

Building a Brain-Healthy Future

Effective public health policies can transform the landscape of Alzheimer's prevention and care. By addressing modifiable risk factors, promoting early detection, and reducing health disparities, these policies can significantly reduce the disease's impact on individuals, families, and societies.

A brain-healthy world is one where prevention is prioritized, resources are equitably distributed, and individuals are empowered to take control of their cognitive health. By investing in policies that support these goals, we take a decisive step toward a future where Alzheimer's is no longer a looming epidemic but a preventable and manageable condition.

Educating the Next Generation

The fight against Alzheimer's disease is not solely about treating current cases—it's about laying the groundwork for a future where the disease can be prevented altogether. Educating the next generation is a cornerstone of this effort, as early awareness and lifelong habits can profoundly shape cognitive health. By empowering young people with knowledge and fostering a culture of brain health, we can create a society that prioritizes prevention and resilience.

The Importance of Early Education

Establishing Lifelong Habits

Many of the behaviors that influence Alzheimer's risk, such as diet, exercise, and sleep, are shaped early in life. Educating children and adolescents about brain health encourages them to adopt habits that protect cognitive function well into old age.

Raising Awareness of Risk Factors

Teaching young people about the relationship between lifestyle choices and brain health helps them understand the importance of preventing conditions like obesity, diabetes, and cardiovascular disease, which are linked to Alzheimer's.

Reducing Stigma

Alzheimer's is often surrounded by stigma and misunderstanding. Early education fosters empathy and awareness, reducing stigma and encouraging open conversations about the disease.

Integrating Brain Health into Education

School Curriculums

Brain Science Basics: Introduce age-appropriate lessons on how the brain works, its role in memory and learning, and how lifestyle choices impact its health.

Healthy Living Classes: Incorporate topics like nutrition, physical activity, sleep hygiene, and stress management into health and physical education programs.

Creative Engagement: Use games, activities, and storytelling to make learning about brain health engaging and memorable for younger students.

Extracurricular Programs

Wellness Clubs: Establish student-led clubs focused on healthy living and cognitive wellness, encouraging peer-to-peer learning and collaboration.

Community Service Projects: Encourage students to volunteer with organizations that support individuals with Alzheimer's, fostering empathy and understanding.

Intergenerational Initiatives

Shared Activities: Pair students with older adults for activities like storytelling, arts and crafts, or technology lessons. These interactions promote mutual learning and highlight the importance of maintaining cognitive engagement throughout life.

Technology and Digital Tools

Leverage apps, games, and online resources that teach brain health concepts in an interactive way. Digital tools can provide engaging ways for young people to track their own healthy habits.

Supporting Families Through Education

Parent and Caregiver Involvement

Provide resources and workshops for parents to reinforce brain-healthy habits at home. Topics might include meal planning, family fitness activities, and strategies for managing stress.

Community Outreach

Partner with schools and community organizations to host events focused on brain health education, ensuring families have access to accurate and actionable information.

Early Family Conversations

Encourage families to discuss Alzheimer's openly, especially if it has affected relatives. Understanding the genetic and lifestyle factors involved can empower young people to take preventive steps.

The Ripple Effect of Education

Cultural Shift

Educating the next generation about brain health fosters a cultural shift where cognitive wellness is a shared priority. This shift encourages systemic changes, such as healthier school meals, improved urban planning for physical activity, and workplace wellness programs.

Future Advocacy

Today's students are tomorrow's leaders. By equipping them with knowledge and a commitment to brain health, we cultivate advocates who can drive research, public health initiatives, and policy changes in the future.

Breaking Cycles of Risk

Early education helps interrupt generational patterns of poor health behaviors, reducing the prevalence of Alzheimer's and other chronic diseases over time.

Building a Brain-Healthy Generation

Educating the next generation is about more than knowledge—it's about instilling a sense of agency and responsibility for their own health and the health of their communities. By teaching young people the importance of brain health and empowering them to take action, we set the stage for a future where Alzheimer's is no longer a pervasive threat.

This investment in education represents a long-term strategy with far-reaching benefits. With informed, proactive young people leading the way, we can envision a society where brain health is a universal priority, and the devastating impacts of Alzheimer's are a thing of the past.

Part IV: The Future of Alzheimer's Research

Chapter 13: Bridging Gaps in Science

What We Still Don't Know

Despite decades of research and significant breakthroughs, Alzheimer's disease remains one of the most complex and challenging conditions to fully understand. While we have made remarkable strides in identifying its hallmarks, such as amyloid plaques and tau tangles, key questions about the disease's root causes, progression, and variability remain unanswered. These gaps in knowledge underscore the need for continued investigation and innovation, as they hold the potential to unlock transformative solutions.

The Unanswered Questions

The True Root Cause

Alzheimer's has long been associated with amyloid-beta and tau pathology, but it is increasingly evident that these are part of a broader network of dysfunctions rather than the sole drivers.

Key Questions:

What initiates the pathological cascade in sporadic Alzheimer's cases?

Are amyloid-beta and tau central causes, or are they downstream effects of other processes, such as mitochondrial dysfunction, neuroinflammation, or vascular damage?

The Role of Inflammation

Chronic neuroinflammation is recognized as a critical component of Alzheimer's, but its exact role—whether as a trigger, a protective response gone awry, or both—remains unclear.

Key Questions:

How does neuroinflammation interact with amyloid and tau pathology?

Can the brain's immune system be modulated to balance protection and repair without exacerbating damage?

The Contribution of Genetics and Epigenetics

Genetic factors such as the APOE4 allele are well-documented, but they do not account for all cases of Alzheimer's, nor do they guarantee disease development.

Key Questions:

What other genetic or epigenetic factors influence risk and progression?

How do environmental exposures and lifestyle choices shape epigenetic modifications in Alzheimer's?

The Role of Non-Neuronal Cells

Microglia, astrocytes, and vascular cells are increasingly recognized as key players in Alzheimer's, but their specific contributions to disease progression are not fully understood.

Key Questions:

How do these cells contribute to the spread of pathology?

Can they be reprogrammed to support repair and recovery?

Why Some Individuals Are Resilient

Cognitive reserve—the brain's ability to compensate for damage—varies widely among individuals. Some people with significant Alzheimer's pathology remain symptom-free, while others experience rapid decline.

Key Questions:

What factors contribute to cognitive resilience?

How can we enhance protective mechanisms to delay or prevent symptom onset?

The Early Stages of the Disease

Alzheimer's begins decades before clinical symptoms appear, but the precise timeline and early mechanisms remain elusive.

Key Questions:

What are the earliest detectable changes in the brain?

How can we develop tools to identify these changes before irreversible damage occurs?

Heterogeneity of the Disease

Alzheimer's does not present uniformly. Some patients experience rapid decline, while others progress slowly or exhibit atypical symptoms.

Key Questions:

What drives the variability in Alzheimer's progression and symptoms?

Are there distinct subtypes of the disease that require different treatment approaches?

Why Treatments Work for Some, but Not Others

Clinical trials have shown mixed results, with some therapies helping certain individuals while failing in others.

Key Questions:

What biomarkers or characteristics predict a patient's response to specific treatments?

How can precision medicine be applied to Alzheimer's to improve outcomes?

Emerging Areas of Exploration

The Gut-Brain Axis

The influence of the gut microbiome on brain health is a burgeoning field, but its exact role in Alzheimer's is still being uncovered.

Systems Biology Approaches

Understanding Alzheimer's as a systems-level disorder involving metabolic, vascular, and immune dysfunctions offers a holistic perspective but requires further study.

Artificial Intelligence in Research

AI tools are being used to analyze complex datasets, identify patterns, and predict disease risk. Their potential to uncover hidden insights is vast but underexplored.

Why These Gaps Matter

Understanding what we still don't know is critical for moving the field forward. These gaps:

Guide Future Research: Prioritizing unanswered questions helps direct funding and effort to areas with the greatest potential impact.

Refine Treatment Strategies: Addressing these unknowns can lead to more targeted and effective therapies.

Empower Prevention Efforts: Identifying early triggers and modifiable risk factors can enable more proactive interventions.

Bridging the Divide

Filling these knowledge gaps requires a multidisciplinary approach, leveraging expertise from fields such as genetics, neuroscience, immunology, and bioinformatics. Collaborative efforts across academic, industry, and government sectors will be essential for accelerating progress.

A Future of Discovery

The mysteries of Alzheimer's challenge us to think beyond established paradigms and embrace innovation. As research continues to evolve, each breakthrough brings us closer to a comprehensive understanding of the disease—an understanding that will pave the way for effective prevention, treatment, and ultimately, a cure.

What we still don't know about Alzheimer's is daunting, but it is also a source of hope and opportunity. By addressing these unanswered questions, we take crucial steps toward unraveling the complexities of the disease and building a future where Alzheimer's no longer holds its devastating grip on humanity.

Collaborative Science and Open-Source Data

The fight against Alzheimer's disease demands a global, collective effort. As the complexity of the disease becomes increasingly evident, the importance of collaboration among researchers, clinicians, and institutions cannot be overstated. Collaborative science and the sharing of open-source data have emerged as transformative approaches, accelerating discoveries, enhancing transparency, and fostering innovation in ways that siloed research cannot achieve.

The Case for Collaboration

The Complexity of Alzheimer's

Alzheimer's is not a single-pathway disease. It involves intricate interactions between genetics, inflammation, vascular health, and lifestyle factors. Collaborative efforts allow researchers from diverse fields to integrate their expertise, creating a more comprehensive understanding of the disease.

Eliminating Redundancy

Duplication of efforts wastes valuable time and resources. Sharing data and methodologies prevents repetition, enabling researchers to build on each other's work rather than starting from scratch.

Access to Diverse Data

Collaborative studies pool data from multiple populations, increasing diversity and enabling insights that are broadly applicable. This is especially important for understanding how Alzheimer's affects different demographic groups.

Faster Translation to Treatment

Collaboration between academic institutions, industry partners, and healthcare providers bridges the gap between basic research and clinical application, speeding the development and deployment of therapies.

The Role of Open-Source Data

Open-source data platforms are revolutionizing Alzheimer's research by providing unrestricted access to datasets, tools, and findings. These platforms democratize research, allowing scientists worldwide to contribute to and benefit from shared knowledge.

Key Open-Source Initiatives

ADNI (Alzheimer's Disease Neuroimaging Initiative): Provides publicly available neuroimaging, genetic, and clinical data to facilitate research on Alzheimer's biomarkers.

AMP-AD (Accelerating Medicines Partnership for Alzheimer's Disease): Offers large-scale, multi-omic datasets, fostering the discovery of therapeutic targets.

UK Biobank and All of Us Research Program: Contain diverse genetic and health data that can be leveraged for Alzheimer's research.

Advancing Machine Learning and AI

Open data is a cornerstone for artificial intelligence in Alzheimer's research. Machine learning algorithms require extensive datasets to identify patterns and generate predictive models. Shared data accelerates these advancements by providing the necessary scale and diversity.

Transparency and Reproducibility

Open data ensures that findings can be validated and replicated, building trust in the scientific process and encouraging robust discoveries.

Challenges in Collaborative Science and Open Data

Data Standardization

Different studies often use varying methodologies, making it difficult to integrate datasets. Establishing universal standards for data collection, storage, and sharing is essential.

Privacy Concerns

Sharing genetic and health data raises concerns about participant privacy and data security. Strong safeguards and anonymization protocols are necessary to protect individuals while enabling research.

Funding and Infrastructure

Collaborative science requires sustained funding and advanced infrastructure, such as high-performance computing and secure data-sharing platforms.

Cultural Barriers

Traditional academic incentives, such as publishing in high-impact journals, may discourage open sharing. Shifting the focus to valuing collaborative contributions is crucial for fostering a culture of openness.

The Benefits of a Collaborative Approach

Accelerated Discovery

Shared data and collective expertise reduce the time needed to identify patterns, test hypotheses, and validate results, bringing us closer to breakthroughs.

Broader Representation

Collaboration across institutions and countries ensures that research includes diverse populations, addressing health disparities and improving the generalizability of findings.

Efficient Resource Use

By pooling resources and expertise, collaborative science maximizes the impact of limited funding and reduces duplication of effort.

Enhanced Innovation

Collaboration sparks creativity and innovation, as researchers from different disciplines share ideas and approaches that might not emerge in isolated efforts.

Looking Ahead: Building a Collaborative Framework

Global Research Consortia

Establish international consortia dedicated to Alzheimer's research, enabling seamless collaboration across borders and institutions.

Incentivizing Data Sharing

Create funding and recognition mechanisms that reward researchers for contributing to open-source platforms and collaborative projects.

Public-Private Partnerships

Foster partnerships between academia, industry, and government to leverage resources, expertise, and infrastructure.

Empowering Citizen Science

Engage the public in Alzheimer's research through initiatives that allow individuals to contribute data, such as cognitive assessments or lifestyle surveys, via apps and online platforms.

A Future United Against Alzheimer's

Collaborative science and open-source data represent a paradigm shift in how we approach Alzheimer's research. By breaking down silos and fostering a culture of transparency and cooperation, we can accelerate progress, ensure inclusivity, and maximize the potential for discovery.

This united approach embodies the essence of tackling a global challenge like Alzheimer's: working together, sharing knowledge, and striving toward a common goal—a world free from the burden of this devastating disease. Through collaboration, we transform not only the trajectory of Alzheimer's but also the way we confront complex medical challenges in the future.

Chapter 14: A Vision for the Future

Toward a World Without Alzheimer's

Imagine a world where Alzheimer's disease no longer robs individuals of their memories, families of their loved ones, and society of its collective wisdom. This vision is not an impossible dream—it is a goal within reach, supported by advancements in science, medicine, and public health. While the road ahead is challenging, the progress made thus far offers hope that we are moving closer to a future where Alzheimer's is preventable, treatable, and ultimately curable.

The Building Blocks of a Cure

Comprehensive Understanding of the Disease

To eliminate Alzheimer's, we must unravel its root causes, progression, and variability. This includes understanding the interplay between genetics, lifestyle, neuroinflammation, and other systemic factors.

Advancing multi-disciplinary research will continue to be crucial in filling the remaining gaps in our knowledge.

Early Detection and Prevention

The earlier we detect Alzheimer's, the better our chances of preventing it. Biomarker technologies, genetic screening, and cognitive testing are paving the way for early intervention strategies that halt the disease before irreversible damage occurs.

Personalized preventative plans will empower individuals to mitigate their unique risk factors, combining cutting-edge tools with lifestyle modifications.

Transformative Treatments

The future of Alzheimer's treatment lies in multi-targeted therapies that address the disease's complexity. Advances in gene therapy, immunotherapy, and pharmacological innovations hold promise for slowing, stopping, or even reversing disease progression.

Lifestyle medicine will complement these medical interventions, ensuring holistic care that promotes overall brain health.

Global Collaboration and Open Science

A world without Alzheimer's will require unprecedented collaboration across nations, disciplines, and sectors. Open-source data sharing, international research consortia, and public-private partnerships will accelerate progress and ensure equitable access to breakthroughs.

Empowered Communities

Education and awareness are essential for building resilient communities. By empowering individuals with knowledge about brain health and fostering supportive environments, we can create a society that prioritizes prevention and care.

The Role of Society

Achieving a world without Alzheimer's is not solely a scientific endeavor—it is a societal commitment. Governments, healthcare systems, and communities must work together to:

Invest in Research and Development: Allocate resources to Alzheimer's research and innovation, ensuring sustained progress.

Improve Healthcare Access: Provide affordable, equitable care, including diagnostics, treatments, and support services, to all individuals regardless of socioeconomic status.

Support Caregivers: Offer robust caregiver training, financial assistance, and respite services to those who shoulder the emotional and physical burden of caregiving.

Promote Brain-Healthy Environments: Create public spaces and policies that encourage physical activity, social connection, and access to nutritious foods.

A Future Defined by Prevention

In this envisioned future, Alzheimer's is no longer an inevitable part of aging. Prevention becomes the norm, with individuals adopting brain-healthy lifestyles from an early age. Routine health checkups include cognitive assessments and biomarker screenings, enabling proactive care that minimizes risk. Communities support brain health through education, wellness programs, and resources that empower people to take charge of their cognitive well-being.

The Impact of a World Without Alzheimer's

The eradication of Alzheimer's would have profound ripple effects:

Improved Quality of Life: Millions of individuals and families would be spared the emotional and financial toll of the disease.

Healthcare Transformation: Freed from the burden of Alzheimer's, healthcare systems could redirect resources toward other pressing challenges.

Economic Benefits: Reduced care costs and the ability of older adults to remain active contributors to society would strengthen economies worldwide.

A Collective Commitment

While a world without Alzheimer's may seem ambitious, the progress made in recent years shows that it is achievable. Advances in research, increasing public awareness, and the dedication of countless scientists, clinicians, and advocates are driving us closer to this goal. However, achieving it will require a collective commitment—from governments and organizations to individuals and families—to prioritize brain health and invest in the future.

A Future of Hope

The vision of a world without Alzheimer's is not just about eradicating a disease—it is about reclaiming the dignity, memories, and lives that Alzheimer's has taken. It is about ensuring that future generations grow old with their cognitive abilities intact, surrounded by the people and memories that define them.

This vision is more than a dream—it is a destination. By continuing to innovate, collaborate, and advocate, we are building the foundation for a future where Alzheimer's is no longer a part of our reality but a challenge we overcame together.

The journey toward a world without Alzheimer's is one of hope, resilience, and determination. Together, we can make this vision a reality.

Expanding the Cure to Other Neurological Diseases

The breakthroughs achieved in Alzheimer's research have the potential to transform our understanding and treatment of other neurological diseases. The intricate mechanisms of Alzheimer's—ranging from amyloid accumulation to neuroinflammation—share commonalities with conditions like Parkinson's disease, Huntington's disease, multiple sclerosis, and even stroke-related cognitive decline. By leveraging the insights and tools developed in the fight against Alzheimer's, we can accelerate progress toward cures for a wide array of brain disorders.

Shared Pathways Across Neurological Diseases

Protein Misfolding and Aggregation

Commonality: Protein misfolding and aggregation are central features of Alzheimer's (amyloid-beta and tau), Parkinson's (alpha-synuclein), and Huntington's (huntingtin protein). These diseases share mechanisms of cellular toxicity and impaired clearance of misfolded proteins.

Potential Advances: Therapies targeting protein aggregation in Alzheimer's, such as monoclonal antibodies, could be adapted to target similar mechanisms in other diseases.

Neuroinflammation

Commonality: Chronic neuroinflammation is a hallmark of many neurodegenerative diseases, including Alzheimer's, Parkinson's, and multiple sclerosis. Overactive immune responses contribute to neuronal damage and disease progression.

Potential Advances: Anti-inflammatory therapies and microglial modulators developed for Alzheimer's may prove effective in mitigating inflammation in other conditions.

Mitochondrial Dysfunction

Commonality: Impaired energy production and oxidative stress are shared features of Alzheimer's, Parkinson's, and amyotrophic lateral sclerosis (ALS).

Potential Advances: Research into enhancing mitochondrial function and reducing oxidative damage in Alzheimer's could benefit a wide range of neurodegenerative diseases.

Synaptic Dysfunction and Neurotransmitter Imbalance

Commonality: Disorders like Alzheimer's, Parkinson's, and schizophrenia involve disruptions in synaptic communication and neurotransmitter systems.

Potential Advances: Alzheimer's treatments aimed at restoring synaptic plasticity and neurotransmitter balance may be repurposed for these conditions.

Cerebrovascular Contributions

Commonality: Vascular dysfunction contributes to Alzheimer's, vascular dementia, and stroke-related cognitive decline.

Potential Advances: Therapies targeting vascular health and blood-brain barrier integrity in Alzheimer's could help prevent and treat cognitive impairments in other vascular-related conditions.

Lessons from Alzheimer's Research

The success of Alzheimer's research provides a roadmap for tackling other neurological diseases:

Biomarker Development

Biomarkers such as amyloid-beta, tau, and neurofilament light chain (NfL) have revolutionized Alzheimer's detection and monitoring. Similar efforts are underway to identify biomarkers for Parkinson's, ALS, and other disorders, enabling earlier diagnosis and tailored treatments.

Precision Medicine

Advances in genetic profiling and personalized approaches to Alzheimer's treatment offer a model for addressing the heterogeneity seen in other neurological diseases.

Therapeutic Platforms

Platforms like CRISPR gene editing, RNA interference, and monoclonal antibodies developed for Alzheimer's can be adapted to target genetic and molecular pathways in other conditions.

Multimodal Therapies

Alzheimer's research has highlighted the need for combination therapies that address multiple pathways simultaneously. This approach can be applied to other complex diseases with multifactorial causes.

The Impact of a Holistic Approach

Expanding the focus of Alzheimer's research to encompass other neurological diseases will yield several benefits:

Accelerated Discovery

Sharing knowledge and resources across disciplines fosters innovation and speeds the development of treatments for multiple conditions.

Reduced Healthcare Burden

Treating common pathways underlying neurological diseases can reduce the overall burden on healthcare systems, improving outcomes for a broad spectrum of patients.

Improved Quality of Life

Advancements in neurological care have the potential to enhance the lives of millions, from individuals with Alzheimer's to those with Parkinson's, ALS, or traumatic brain injury.

Challenges and Opportunities

Disease-Specific Variability

While neurological diseases share common pathways, each has unique features that require tailored interventions. Research must strike a balance between broad applicability and disease-specific precision.

Resource Allocation

Expanding the focus to include multiple diseases may stretch funding and resources. Collaborative funding models and public-private partnerships can help address this challenge.

Ethical Considerations

As research expands, ethical concerns about data sharing, trial participation, and access to treatments must be carefully managed.

The Vision of a Unified Approach

The ultimate goal is to create a unified framework for understanding and treating neurological diseases. By integrating insights from Alzheimer's research with discoveries in related fields, we can develop therapies that address the brain's interconnected systems rather than isolated conditions.

A Future of Shared Progress

The breakthroughs achieved in Alzheimer's research have already illuminated pathways that extend beyond a single disease. By expanding this knowledge to encompass other neurological disorders, we take a significant step toward a future where brain health is comprehensively understood and protected.

This shared progress underscores the interconnectedness of science, reminding us that advances in one area can reverberate across many. Together, we can envision a world where Alzheimer's and other neurological diseases no longer define the future of aging but instead serve as challenges we have overcome through innovation, collaboration, and determination.

Conclusion

Why This Matters for Humanity

Alzheimer's disease is more than a medical condition—it is a profound human challenge that affects individuals, families, and societies in deeply personal and far-reaching ways. It steals memories, dismantles identities, and places an emotional and economic burden on caregivers and communities. Yet, it also unites us in a shared mission to understand, prevent, and one day cure this devastating disease.

The journey to conquer Alzheimer's is not just about solving a scientific puzzle—it's about reaffirming our humanity, our interconnectedness, and our capacity for resilience and innovation. The fight against Alzheimer's matters because it touches the essence of what it means to be human: our memories, our relationships, and our ability to live meaningful lives.

Protecting the Fabric of Identity

Memory is the foundation of identity. It holds the stories of who we are, where we've been, and who we love. Alzheimer's robs individuals of this vital connection to themselves and others, creating a profound loss that extends beyond the individual to their family and community. Every advance in understanding and treating Alzheimer's is a step toward preserving the dignity and identity of millions of people worldwide.

Empowering Families and Caregivers

The impact of Alzheimer's ripples through families, testing their emotional and financial resilience. Caregivers bear the weight of the disease, often sacrificing their own health and well-being to care for loved ones. By advancing prevention, early detection, and treatment, we can ease this burden, offering families hope and the tools to navigate Alzheimer's with strength and support.

Strengthening Societies

Alzheimer's is a global challenge that transcends borders, affecting people of all races, ethnicities, and socioeconomic statuses. As the global population ages, the prevalence of Alzheimer's threatens to overwhelm healthcare systems and economies. Investing in research, education, and public health initiatives is not just a moral imperative—it is essential for creating sustainable, equitable societies capable of addressing the challenges of an aging world.

A Testament to Human Ingenuity

The effort to unravel Alzheimer's is a testament to the power of human ingenuity. It showcases our ability to tackle complex problems, adapt to new discoveries, and collaborate across disciplines and nations. Every breakthrough reflects the collective efforts of researchers, clinicians, caregivers, and advocates who refuse to accept the inevitability of this disease.

A Shared Hope for the Future

The fight against Alzheimer's is about more than curing a disease—it is about imagining a better future. A future where aging is no longer feared but embraced as a time of wisdom and reflection. A future where individuals and families are spared the pain of watching their loved ones fade away. A future where our shared humanity is strengthened by the knowledge that we can overcome even the most daunting challenges together.

Why This Matters

This matters because Alzheimer's is not just a disease of the brain—it is a disease of the human experience. It matters because every life touched by Alzheimer's holds value, and every effort to combat the disease brings us closer to honoring that value. It matters because the fight against Alzheimer's is ultimately a fight for our shared humanity.

The journey to a world without Alzheimer's is not merely a scientific endeavor—it is a deeply human one. By embracing innovation, compassion, and collaboration, we are not just addressing a disease; we are shaping the future of humanity. Together, we can ensure that Alzheimer's becomes a story of the past, a challenge we overcame, and a reminder of the strength and resilience that define us as human beings.

A Call to Action

The fight against Alzheimer's disease is not one that can be won by researchers and healthcare professionals alone—it requires the collective effort of individuals, families, communities, and governments. Alzheimer's affects us all, whether directly or indirectly, and the challenge it poses demands a response that is as collaborative as it is urgent. The advances we've made in understanding and addressing Alzheimer's are remarkable, but the road ahead remains long, and we cannot afford complacency.

Why We Must Act

The Growing Impact

With Alzheimer's cases projected to triple by 2050, the time to act is now. This disease places an immense emotional, financial, and societal burden on families and healthcare systems worldwide. Delaying action will only compound these challenges.

The Potential for Progress

We are on the brink of breakthroughs. Advances in biomarker detection, personalized medicine, and therapeutic innovations have brought us closer than ever to effective prevention and treatment. Every investment in Alzheimer's research moves us closer to the day when this disease is no longer a threat.

The Human Cost

Behind every statistic is a person—a parent, grandparent, sibling, or friend—whose life is altered by Alzheimer's. Their struggles remind us that this fight is not abstract; it is deeply personal, affecting the very core of human relationships and identity.

How You Can Make a Difference

Educate Yourself and Others

Knowledge is power. Understanding the risk factors, early signs, and prevention strategies for Alzheimer's empowers individuals to take proactive steps for their own brain health and that of their loved ones.

Support Research and Advocacy

Whether through donating to Alzheimer's research organizations, participating in clinical trials, or advocating for increased funding and resources, your support fuels progress. Every contribution brings us closer to a cure.

Foster a Brain-Healthy Lifestyle

Adopt and encourage habits that promote cognitive health, such as regular exercise, a nutritious diet, quality sleep, and social engagement. Small changes can have a big impact, especially when embraced collectively.

Champion Caregiver Support

Caregivers are the unsung heroes in the fight against Alzheimer's. Advocate for policies that provide them with resources, respite care, and financial support. Volunteer with organizations that assist caregivers and families affected by Alzheimer's.

Engage Your Community

Build awareness within your community through events, workshops, or support groups. A strong, informed community is better equipped to support individuals and families affected by the disease.

Demand Policy Action

Call on policymakers to prioritize Alzheimer's research and healthcare initiatives. Advocate for equitable access to diagnostics, treatments, and care for all individuals, regardless of socioeconomic status.

The Power of Collective Action

Alzheimer's is a global challenge that requires a global response. By uniting our efforts—across borders, disciplines, and generations—we can transform the future of this disease. Together, we have the power to:

Prevent Alzheimer's through education and lifestyle changes.

Detect the disease early with accessible tools and technologies.

Develop effective treatments that slow, stop, or reverse its progression.

Build a world where individuals and families no longer fear the loss of memory, identity, and connection.

A Legacy of Hope

Your actions today can shape the world of tomorrow. By committing to the fight against Alzheimer's, you contribute to a legacy of hope—a world where future generations grow old with their memories intact, their relationships preserved, and their lives enriched by the knowledge that we faced this challenge and triumphed.

Join the Movement

This is a call to action for every person who has been touched by Alzheimer's, for every community striving for health and resilience, and for every leader with the power to make a difference. Together, we can achieve what once seemed impossible: a world without Alzheimer's.

The time to act is now. The fight is ours. And the future is bright with the promise of what we can achieve when we stand united against Alzheimer's disease.

Appendices

Glossary of Terms

This glossary provides definitions for key terms and concepts discussed in *Unraveling Alzheimer's: The Definitive Guide to Its Cause and Cure*. These definitions aim to enhance understanding and provide clarity for readers exploring the complex subject of Alzheimer's disease.

A

Amyloid-Beta (Aβ): A protein fragment that aggregates to form plaques in the brain, a hallmark of Alzheimer's disease.

Amyloid Plaques: Clumps of amyloid-beta protein that accumulate between neurons, disrupting communication and contributing to neurodegeneration.

Antioxidants: Molecules that prevent oxidative damage by neutralizing free radicals, supporting cellular health and reducing inflammation.

APOE (Apolipoprotein E): A gene that plays a role in lipid metabolism. The APOE4 variant is the strongest genetic risk factor for late-onset Alzheimer's.

B

Biomarkers: Biological indicators, such as proteins or imaging findings, used to detect or monitor a disease. In Alzheimer's, common biomarkers include amyloid-beta, tau, and neurofilament light chain.

Brain-Derived Neurotrophic Factor (BDNF): A protein that supports neuron survival, growth, and synaptic plasticity, essential for memory and learning.

C

Cerebrospinal Fluid (CSF): A clear fluid surrounding the brain and spinal cord, often analyzed for biomarkers like amyloid-beta and tau to diagnose Alzheimer's.

Cognitive Reserve: The brain's ability to adapt and compensate for damage, delaying the onset of Alzheimer's symptoms despite pathology.

Cognitive Decline: The gradual loss of cognitive functions such as memory, attention, and reasoning, often associated with aging or neurodegenerative diseases.

D

Dementia: A general term for a decline in cognitive function severe enough to interfere with daily life. Alzheimer's disease is the most common cause of dementia.

Diagnostics: Tools and tests used to identify Alzheimer's, including biomarker assays, neuroimaging, and cognitive assessments.

E

Early-Onset Alzheimer's: A rare form of Alzheimer's that develops before age 65, often linked to genetic mutations.

Epigenetics: Changes in gene expression caused by environmental and lifestyle factors rather than alterations in the DNA sequence itself.

G

Gene Therapy: A treatment approach that modifies or repairs genes to address the root causes of diseases, including Alzheimer's.

Glymphatic System: The brain's waste clearance system, active primarily during sleep, which removes toxins such as amyloid-beta.

H

Hippocampus: A brain region critical for memory and learning, often one of the first areas affected by Alzheimer's.

Hyperphosphorylated Tau: A form of tau protein that becomes abnormal and aggregates into tangles, contributing to Alzheimer's pathology.

I

Inflammation: The immune system's response to injury or infection. Chronic neuroinflammation is a key factor in Alzheimer's progression.

Insulin Resistance: A metabolic condition linked to impaired glucose metabolism, associated with an increased risk of Alzheimer's.

M

Microglia: Immune cells in the brain that help clear debris and toxins. Overactivation of microglia contributes to neuroinflammation in Alzheimer's.

Mitochondrial Dysfunction: Impaired function of mitochondria, the cell's energy producers, leading to oxidative stress and contributing to Alzheimer's pathology.

N

Neurodegeneration: The progressive loss of structure or function of neurons, leading to cognitive and functional decline.

Neurofibrillary Tangles: Twisted fibers of hyperphosphorylated tau protein found inside neurons, disrupting their function in Alzheimer's.

Neuroinflammation: Inflammation within the brain, often caused by overactivation of the immune system in response to Alzheimer's pathology.

Neuroplasticity: The brain's ability to reorganize itself by forming new neural connections, a critical factor in cognitive resilience.

P

Precision Medicine: A tailored approach to treatment that considers an individual's genetic, environmental, and lifestyle factors.

Proteopathy: A disease caused by abnormal protein folding and aggregation, such as Alzheimer's (amyloid-beta and tau) and Parkinson's (alpha-synuclein).

S

Short-Chain Fatty Acids (SCFAs): Compounds produced by gut bacteria that have anti-inflammatory and neuroprotective effects.

Sleep Hygiene: Habits and practices that promote quality sleep, essential for glymphatic function and brain health.

Sporadic Alzheimer's: The most common form of Alzheimer's, with no clear genetic cause, typically developing after age 65.

T

Tau Protein: A protein involved in stabilizing microtubules in neurons. In Alzheimer's, tau becomes abnormal and forms tangles that impair neuron function.

TREM2 (Triggering Receptor Expressed on Myeloid Cells 2): A receptor on microglia that regulates immune responses. Mutations in TREM2 are linked to an increased risk of Alzheimer's.

V

Vascular Contributions to Cognitive Impairment and Dementia (VCID): Cognitive decline caused or exacerbated by vascular problems, often coexisting with Alzheimer's.

Vagus Nerve: A cranial nerve involved in regulating inflammation and brain-gut communication, relevant to Alzheimer's and other neurological conditions.

W

Wearable Technology: Devices that monitor health metrics, such as physical activity, sleep, and cognitive function, aiding in early detection and management of Alzheimer's.

This glossary is designed to serve as a resource for readers to navigate the complex terminology associated with Alzheimer's disease and related topics. Understanding these terms is a step toward empowering individuals to engage with the science and contribute to the collective effort to combat Alzheimer's.

Summary of Key Studies

This section summarizes pivotal studies that have shaped our understanding of Alzheimer's disease, its causes, and potential treatments. These studies highlight breakthroughs in genetics, biomarkers, pathology, and interventions, offering a foundation for current and future research.

1. Discovery of Alzheimer's Disease (1906)

Study: Alois Alzheimer's Identification of Plaques and Tangles

Key Findings:

Alois Alzheimer first described the disease in a patient with severe memory loss and behavioral changes. Post-mortem examination revealed amyloid plaques and neurofibrillary tangles in the brain, establishing the pathological hallmarks of the condition.

Significance:
Provided the foundation for understanding Alzheimer's as a distinct neurodegenerative disease.

2. Framingham Heart Study (1948–Present)

Focus: Cardiovascular Health and Cognitive Decline

Key Findings:

Longitudinal data demonstrated the link between cardiovascular risk factors (e.g., hypertension, diabetes) and the increased risk of Alzheimer's.

Significance:

Highlighted the importance of vascular health in preventing cognitive decline and Alzheimer's.

3. Genetics of Alzheimer's Disease (1993)

Study: Discovery of the APOE4 Gene Variant

Key Findings:

Researchers identified the APOE4 allele as the strongest genetic risk factor for late-onset Alzheimer's.

Significance:
Revolutionized genetic research in Alzheimer's, enabling risk stratification and personalized approaches to prevention and treatment.

4. Alzheimer's Disease Neuroimaging Initiative (ADNI) (2004–Present)

Focus: Biomarkers for Early Detection

Key Findings:

Established standardized protocols for imaging and biomarker analysis, including amyloid and tau PET imaging, CSF biomarkers, and structural MRI.

Significance:
Enabled early detection and monitoring of disease progression, facilitating clinical trials for new therapies.

5. Accelerating Medicines Partnership for Alzheimer's Disease (AMP-AD) (2014–Present)

Focus: Multi-Omic Data Sharing

Key Findings:

Developed open-access datasets integrating genomics,

proteomics, and transcriptomics to identify new therapeutic targets.

Significance:
Accelerated the discovery of potential drug candidates and highlighted the role of systems biology in Alzheimer's research.

---

6. Anti-Amyloid Therapy Trials (2016–2023)

Studies: Aducanumab, Lecanemab, and Donanemab Trials

Key Findings:

Monoclonal antibodies targeting amyloid-beta demonstrated modest reductions in amyloid plaques and slowed cognitive decline in some patients with early-stage Alzheimer's.

Significance:
Marked a turning point in therapeutic development, validating the amyloid hypothesis while highlighting the need for multimodal treatments.

---

7. Lifestyle and Cognitive Decline: FINGER Study (2015)

Focus: Lifestyle Interventions in Aging Populations

Key Findings:

The Finnish Geriatric Intervention Study to Prevent Cognitive Impairment and Disability (FINGER) demonstrated that a combination of diet, exercise, cognitive training, and vascular risk monitoring improved cognitive performance in at-risk older adults.

Significance:
Established lifestyle interventions as a cornerstone of Alzheimer's prevention strategies.

---

8. Role of Neuroinflammation: TREM2 Research (2017)

Focus: Microglial Function in Alzheimer's

Key Findings:

Studies revealed that mutations in the TREM2 gene impair microglial function, leading to insufficient clearance of amyloid plaques and increased neuroinflammation.

Significance:
Highlighted the critical role of the brain's immune system in Alzheimer's progression and opened new avenues for immunomodulatory therapies.

9. Gut-Brain Axis Research (2018–Present)

Focus: Microbiome and Cognitive Health

Key Findings:

Studies demonstrated links between gut dysbiosis, systemic inflammation, and Alzheimer's pathology.

Significance:
Suggested that modifying the gut microbiome through diet, probiotics, or fecal microbiota transplantation could influence brain health.

10. CRISPR and Gene Therapy Advances (2019–Present)

Focus: Targeted Gene Editing for Alzheimer's

Key Findings:

Preclinical studies using CRISPR-Cas9 showed potential for silencing genes involved in amyloid-beta production and neuroinflammation.

Significance:
Opened the door to precise genetic interventions for Alzheimer's and related conditions.

11. Sleep and Glymphatic Research (2020)

Focus: Sleep-Driven Clearance of Amyloid-Beta

Key Findings:

Identified the glymphatic system's role in clearing amyloid-beta during deep sleep. Sleep disturbances were linked to increased amyloid accumulation.

Significance:
Highlighted sleep optimization as a key preventive strategy for Alzheimer's.

12. Digital Biomarkers for Alzheimer's (2022–Present)

Focus: Wearable and App-Based Monitoring

Key Findings:

Emerging technologies demonstrated the feasibility of detecting subtle cognitive and behavioral changes indicative of early Alzheimer's.

Significance:
Provided scalable, non-invasive tools for widespread screening and early intervention.

Conclusion

These landmark studies reflect the evolution of Alzheimer's research, from its initial discovery to cutting-edge advancements in genetics, biomarkers, and treatment. Each study has contributed a piece to the puzzle, bringing us closer to understanding, preventing, and ultimately curing this devastating disease. The lessons from these studies underscore the importance of collaboration, innovation, and continued investment in Alzheimer's research.

Practical Guides for Caregivers and Patients

Caring for someone with Alzheimer's disease is a challenging yet deeply meaningful journey. This section provides practical advice for caregivers and patients to navigate the complexities of Alzheimer's while maintaining quality of life. These guides cover essential topics, from daily caregiving strategies to fostering emotional well-being and preparing for future needs.

1. For Caregivers

Building a Support System

Involve Family and Friends: Don't hesitate to ask for help. Assign specific tasks to trusted family members and friends, such as running errands, preparing meals, or providing respite care.

Join Support Groups: Sharing experiences with other caregivers can provide emotional support and practical advice. Local and online groups are available through organizations like the Alzheimer's Association.

Leverage Community Resources: Look into adult daycare programs, in-home care services, and respite care options to lighten your load.

Establishing Routines

Consistency is Key: Maintain a regular daily schedule to reduce confusion and anxiety for the person with Alzheimer's.

Simplify Activities: Break tasks into manageable steps and offer gentle guidance as needed. For example, when dressing, lay out clothing in the order it should be put on.

Communicating Effectively

Stay Patient and Calm: Speak slowly, use simple sentences, and maintain a positive tone.

Nonverbal Cues Matter: A smile, touch, or reassuring gesture can often communicate more effectively than words.

Redirect Instead of Correcting: If the person becomes confused or upset, gently redirect their focus to something calming rather than correcting them.

Managing Behavioral Challenges

Identify Triggers: Keep a journal to identify patterns or situations that cause agitation or aggression.

Use Redirection: Distract the person with a favorite activity or soothing music when they become upset.

Maintain a Calm Environment: Reduce noise, clutter, and distractions to minimize confusion.

Taking Care of Yourself

Prioritize Your Health: Eat well, exercise, and get enough rest.

Set Boundaries: Learn to say no to nonessential tasks to avoid burnout.

Seek Professional Help: Consider counseling or therapy to process the emotional challenges of caregiving.

---

2. For Patients

Maintaining Cognitive Health

Engage in Brain-Boosting Activities: Play puzzles, read, or participate in hobbies you enjoy to stimulate your mind.

Stay Socially Connected: Spend time with loved ones, join a club, or volunteer to maintain emotional and cognitive engagement.

Adopt a Healthy Lifestyle: Eat a balanced diet, exercise regularly, and prioritize quality sleep.

Planning for the Future

Legal and Financial Planning: Work with an attorney or financial planner to establish powers of attorney, advance directives, and estate planning while you are still able to make decisions.

Discuss Care Preferences: Share your wishes for future care with family members to ensure they understand your preferences.

Consider Clinical Trials: Explore participation in clinical trials, which can provide access to cutting-edge treatments and contribute to research efforts.

Managing Emotions

Acknowledge Your Feelings: It's natural to feel frustration, sadness, or fear. Talking to a trusted friend, therapist, or support group can help.

Practice Stress Reduction: Techniques such as mindfulness, yoga, or meditation can help manage anxiety and improve well-being.

Celebrate Small Wins: Focus on what you can still do rather than what you have lost. Celebrate moments of joy and connection.

---

3. Home Safety Tips

Minimize Fall Risks: Remove clutter, secure loose rugs, and install grab bars in bathrooms.

Label and Organize: Use clear labels on drawers, cabinets, and appliances to help the person locate items easily.

Secure Hazardous Items: Keep medications, cleaning supplies, and sharp objects locked away.

Wander Prevention: Install locks on doors and consider a GPS tracker for individuals prone to wandering.

---

4. Preparing for Advanced Stages

Transitioning to Professional Care: Explore memory care facilities or in-home nursing options early to make informed decisions.

End-of-Life Planning: Discuss hospice care and palliative options to ensure comfort and dignity in the final stages.

Legacy and Connection: Encourage the person to record memories, write letters, or create photo albums for loved ones to cherish.

5. Technology Tools for Support

Memory Aids: Use apps or devices that provide reminders for medications, appointments, or daily tasks.

Safety Monitoring: Install motion sensors, cameras, or GPS trackers for enhanced safety and peace of mind.

Communication Tools: Video calling apps and photo-sharing platforms can help patients stay connected with loved ones.

6. Resources for Caregivers and Patients

Alzheimer's Association (alz.org): Comprehensive support, resources, and a 24/7 helpline for caregivers and patients.

Local Aging Agencies: Contact your area's agency on aging for information on services, programs, and financial assistance.

Books and Guides: Explore caregiver handbooks and Alzheimer's care guides for in-depth advice and strategies.

This guide is designed to offer practical, actionable advice for managing the daily realities of Alzheimer's disease. By empowering caregivers and patients with the tools and resources they need, we can foster resilience, maintain dignity, and create moments of connection and joy throughout the journey.

www.ingramcontent.com/pod-product-compliance
Lightning Source LLC
Chambersburg PA
CBHW052206220526
45471CB00004B/1842